The Nutrition Twins
Veggie Cure

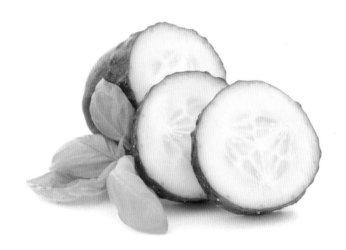

Expert Advice and Tantalizing Recipes
for Health, Energy, and Beauty

The Nutrition Twins:
Lyssie Lakatos, RD, CDN, CFT,
and Tammy Lakatos Shames, RD, CDN, CFT

skirt!

Guilford, Connecticut
An imprint of Globe Pequot Press

TO SUMMER AND RILEY

To buy books in quantity for corporate use
or incentives, call **(800) 962-0973**
or e-mail **premiums@GlobePequot.com**.

 skirt!® is an attitude . . . spirited, independent, outspoken, serious, playful and irreverent, sometimes controversial, always passionate.

skirt!® is an imprint of Globe Pequot Press.
skirt!® is a registered trademark of Morris Publishing Group, LLC, and is used with express permission.

All photos in Part I and on pp. i, viii, 101, 105, 108, 109, 110 ,111, 115, 116, 121, 134, 145, 150, 151, 153, 155, 180, 183, 184, 193, 201, 211, 215, 227, 228, 231, 234, 235, and 239 licensed by Shutterstock.com.
All other recipe photos by Ron Manville.

Text design: Sheryl Pirolo Kober
Layout artist: Melissa Evarts
Project editors: David Legere and Meredith Dias

Library of Congress Cataloging-in-Publication Data

Shames, Tammy Lakatos.
The nutrition twins' veggie cure : expert advice and tantalizing recipes for health, energy, and beauty / Tammy Lakatos Shames, RD, CDN, CFT, and Lyssie Lakatos, RD, CDN, CFT.
pages cm
Summary: "The Nutrition Twins, Tammy Lakatos Shames and Lyssie Lakatos, both registered dietitians, reveal the vegetables that help specific health problems, and provide 100-plus delicious and nutritious recipes to put this "cure" immediately in action on your plate. Includes an easy to follow menu plan for a 10-day Jumpstart to Health and Weight Loss"— Provided by publisher.
ISBN 978-0-7627-8476-9 (pbk.)
1. Vegetarianism. 2. Vegan cooking. Veganism. 3. Cooking for the sick.
I. Lakatos, Lyssie. II. Title.
RM236.S53 2013
641.5'636—dc23
2013015026

Printed in the United States of America

10 9 8 7 6 5 4 3 2 1

Contents

Introduction vi

PART I: VEGGIES FOR YOUR HEALTH AND WELL-BEING

Chapter 1: Stress Relieving and Tension Taming: Veggies to Take the Edge Off 2
   Spotlight on:
      Summer Squash 3
      Green Beans 5

Chapter 2: Beat the Bloat and Clean the Pipes: Veggies for Belly Relief 8
   Spotlight on:
      Fennel 9
      Artichokes 11

Chapter 3: I Heart My Veggies: Veggies That Keep Your
            Cardiovascular System in Tune 13
   Spotlight on:
      Black Beans 17
      Crimini Mushrooms 19
      Swiss Chard 21
      Garlic 23

Chapter 4: Crunching against Cancer: Veggies That Help Reduce Risk 26
   Spotlight on:
      Onions 26
      Brussels Sprouts 29

Chapter 5: Bone Boosting Bonanzas: Veggie Recipes Built to Build Strong Bones 31
   Spotlight on:
      Peas 34
      Turnip Greens 36

Chapter 6: The Slim & Trim Factor: Veggies to Lose Weight Fast 39
   Spotlight on:
      Cabbage (Green, Red, Savoy) and Bok Choy 39
      Celery 42

Contents

Chapter 7: The Perk-Up Factor: Veggies for Energy   44
    Spotlight on:
      Butternut Squash 44
      Potatoes 47

Chapter 8: Skin Dulgence: Veggies That Are Better than Anti-Wrinkle Cream   50
    Spotlight on:
      Tomatoes. 50
      Cucumbers 52

Chapter 9: A Bun (Loaded with Veggies) in the Oven: Veggies
    for a Healthy Pregnancy   55
    Spotlight on:
      Asparagus 55
      Romaine Lettuce 57

Chapter 10: I Don't Have Time: Veggies for When You've Only Got Five Minutes 60
    Spotlight on:
      Cauliflower 60
      Spinach 62

Chapter 11: Mood-Boosting Must-Haves: Veggies That Lift Your Spirit   65
    Spotlight on:
      Sweet Potatoes 66
      Spaghetti Squash 68

Chapter 12: Hunger Games: Veggies You Can Sink Your Teeth Into   71
    Spotlight on:
      Eggplant 71
      Portobello Mushrooms. 73

Chapter 13: Detox and Cleanse: Veggies That Flush Toxins after Overindulgence 75
    Spotlight on:
      Beets 76
      Kale 79

Chapter 14: Salad Haters' Delights: Veggies for Irresistible Bowl Creations 81
    Spotlight on:
      Corn 82
      Olives 84

Chapter 15:   My Kid Won't Eat Veggies: Veggies Kids Will Love   87
    Spotlight on:
      Broccoli 89
      Carrots. 91

Chapter 16:   More Bang per Bite: Veggie Duos That Enhance Nutrient Absorption 93
    Spotlight on:
      Avocados 96
      Bell Peppers 98

PART II: RECIPES

Chapter 17:   The Nutrition Twins' Veggie Cure Recipes   102
    Legend 105
    Breakfasts and Smoothies 106
    Appetizers and Snacks 126
    Soups and Salads 159
    Mains 185
    Sides 205

10-Day Weight Loss Jumpstart, Belly De-Bloat, and Toxin Flush. 240

Metric Conversion Tables. 247

Acknowledgments 248

Recipe Index 250

Index 252

Introduction

We admit it, even we—the Nutrition Twins, registered dietitians and personal trainers who live, breathe, and coach good health for a living—haven't always loved our vegetables. Today we down our veggies like nobody's business. Why the change of heart?

Well, after years of nutrition education and observing firsthand how vegetables make your skin glow and your hair shine, and help keep you lean and fit while boosting your energy and fighting practically every physical ailment, we learned to like them. We're now among the fortunate who truly love their veggies. We love them so much, in fact, that we like our veggies served with a side of . . . veggies. Brussels sprouts with broccoli, tomatoes with eggplant, kale with leeks, spinach with mushrooms—you name it, we're fans, and our mouths are already watering.

We do realize this is rare. Most people don't enjoy their veggies in such quantities and served just plain the way we do. Knowing that vegetables help keep them healthy encourages some people to nibble on a salad here or there, but most need a little (or a lot of) extra flavor to eat even close to the recommended daily amounts. Americans are missing the mark so severely when it comes to meeting their bodies' vegetable requirements that the United States Department of Agriculture decided it needed to step in and make the message clear. In 2011 the USDA created MyPlate, a simple visual cue that depicts how you should eat to be healthy and shows that you should "make half your plate fruits and vegetables." Although that includes fruits, experts agree the majority of that side of the plate should come from veggies.

Because we've made the change ourselves and experienced the rewards, we want to help you fill that half of your plate. We want everyone to feel motivated by their quest for good health, by their taste buds—even by vanity!—to eat their vegetables. After witnessing thousands of our clients as well as ourselves personally reap the "fruits" of vegetable consumption, we feel it's our mission to help everyone to feel and look as good as they deserve. That's why we've written this book. We've got foolproof ways to ensure that everyone (this includes you) will meet their veggie needs. We've got the recipes that will get you hooked on veggies so that you can change your life for the better—and for good. Our recipes are so scrumptious that even those with the pickiest of palates will be satisfied.

If cancer, heart disease, or high blood pressure runs in your family, we share simple secrets for getting the best veggies to lower your risk of these diseases while tantalizing your taste buds. If you long to fight wrinkles and aging, we provide easy, delicious ways to keep your skin—and your body—youthful. If you strive to feel better, happier, and more energetic, we've got your veggie prescription and the recipe to fill it while seducing your palate. And if you need a plant-based mood booster, a quick slim-down a week before your wedding, repair for your skin and age spots without the laser, or even just a surge of energy, then look no further—we have the veggie cures for you. What's more, if your goal is to lose weight, we've got veggies you can sink your teeth into, veggie "detox" recipes to remedy the damage done after a long night, and veggies that will give your body a massage from the inside out.

If you avoid veggies because you don't think they taste good or you simply aren't excited to eat them, then you need to try these recipes—they're formulated just for you: someone who needs to be wowed by their veggies. If you give veggies the cold shoulder because you don't have the time to prepare them, we've created recipes for you that are super easy to whip together and so delicious that you'd likely make them even if they took longer to prepare.

Altogether we've created more than 100 scrumptious veggie recipes, tested them, and analyzed the nutrition content to ensure that you have the perfect recipes to match your prescription. Simply use our Veggie Cure as your bible to get you what you want—it's your veggie prescription to meet your personal goals.

All the work has been done for you. Just pick a health, energy, or beauty goal and you'll be on your way to achieving it. That's because we've laid out the book so that you can go directly to the chapter that addresses your goal. In that chapter you'll find your veggie prescription—the vegetables that will give you what you want—and we tell you why those vegetables work their magic. We also highlight several vegetable superstars. Then we give you the recipes that correspond to your veggie prescription. For example, if you frequently feel bloated and want to flush all of that puffiness that your body is holding, you'll turn to chapter 2, "Beat the Bloat and Clean the Pipes," and you'll find the vegetables that will do the work for you. You'll see why certain vegetables will get rid of those swollen fingers and belly. You'll then learn about the spotlighted anti-bloat veggies, fennel and artichokes, and be directed to specific recipes to make. You'll see options like Fennel Stuffed Potatoes, Golden Gazpacho in Petite Cucumber Cradles, Roasted Fennel, Rockin' Ratatouille, Tomato Artichoke Pasta Bake, Artichoke Hummus, and Parmesan Baked Artichoke and their complete recipes in the back of the book. Choose a recipe, give it a try, and you'll be well on your way to a flat stomach and puff-free eyes. We provide this "cure" for whatever ails you!

Regardless of your goal or which chapter you turn to first, this book takes you by the hand, guiding you step by step to a better, happier, healthier you. We can't wait for you to reap the benefits of the Veggie Cure!

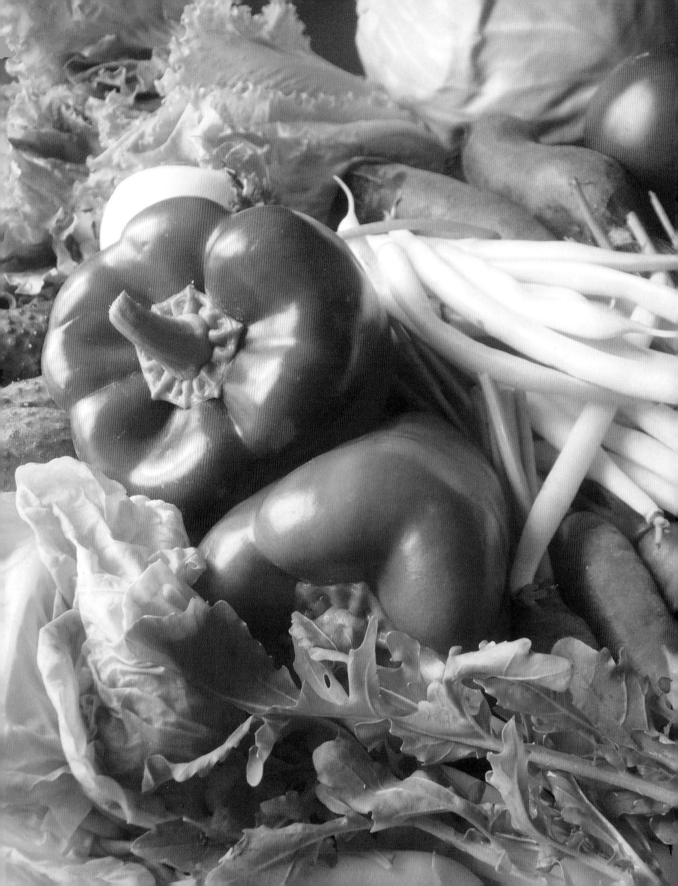

PART I

veggies for your health and well-being

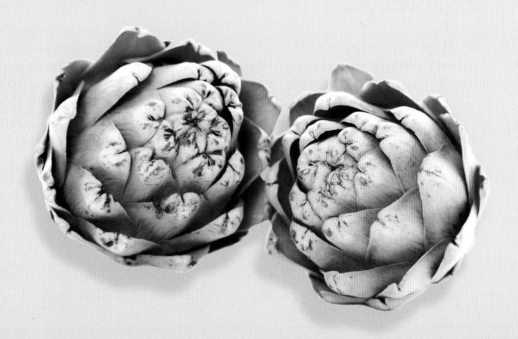

CHAPTER 1

Stress Relieving and Tension Taming

Veggies to Take the Edge Off

The Problem: You feel the stress of everyday life is starting to catch up with you, triggering cravings and stress eating, causing you to lose sleep, making you moody, and speeding the aging process inside your body and out—creating fine lines and bags under your eyes. You don't want stress to get the best of you.

Here's What You Need: All vegetables! Particularly mushrooms, leafy greens, squash, potatoes, bell peppers, spinach, bok choy, fennel, string beans, edamame, and others that are good sources of magnesium, vitamin B_6, vitamin C, potassium, copper, calcium, and omega-3s, as well as folate (folic acid), other B vitamins, and tryptophan.

Here's Why: While certain foods contain nutrients that the body uses to tame stress, vegetables have a leg up, as they also contain fiber to help stabilize energy levels and prevent mood swings. This is essential to better cope with stress and to prevent cravings and the subsequent overeating associated with it. Nutrients like calcium and vitamin C are quickly depleted during stress. Omega-3 fatty acids, folic acid, and other B vitamins fight anxiety and depression and

help provide an overstressed body with energy. Several nutrients like tryptophan and omega-3 fatty acids are needed to make the feel-good/relaxation brain chemical serotonin. Potassium and magnesium calm you on the inside as they relax your blood vessels and your muscles, keeping blood pressure down, keeping your arteries pliable, and helping your blood flow freely so that stress-reducing nutrients can easily be delivered throughout your body.

Here's How to Get It: Vitamin C is plentiful in tomatoes, cucumbers, bell peppers, broccoli, and potatoes. Go for dark leafy greens—collard greens, turnip greens, kale, spinach, bok choy (also known as Chinese cabbage), dandelion greens, mustard greens, parsley, watercress—and broccoli and beans for calcium. Just $2\frac{1}{4}$ cups of cooked broccoli provide as much calcium as a cup of milk, and you can also get calcium from soybeans and tofu. Omega-3s are found in cabbage, kale, green beans, and summer squash. Get folic acid and B vitamins from asparagus, soybeans, sweet potatoes, spinach, and lettuce. Your best potassium bets? Tomato products, potatoes, spinach, and sweet potatoes—so bite into our Fennel Stuffed Potatoes (page 189). For magnesium reach for beans, especially pinto, black, white, and kidney beans. Also get it from spinach, beet greens, okra, tomato products, artichokes, plantains, potatoes, sweet potatoes, and collard greens.

Are you taking common medications like anti-inflammatory drugs, cholesterol-lowering drugs, birth control pills, or diabetes medications? They can deplete your body's folate (folic acid) supply, so be extra sure to get enough folate.

Spotlight on Summer Squash

Recipes with Summer Squash (Zucchini): Carrot Zucchini Muffins, page 128; Cream of Whatever Soup, page 159; Dieter's Delight Chock Full of Veggies Soup, page 163; Fennel Stuffed Potatoes, page 189; Heavenly Roasted Vegetables, page 219; Mediterranean Pizza, page 192; Rockin' Ratatouille, page 152; Teriyaki-Lime Veggie and Pineapple Kebabs, page 237; Vegetable Ribbons, page 239; Veggie Frittata Bites, page 121; Zucchini Canoes, page 158; Zucchini Fritters, page 124, Zucchinilicious Lasagna, page 204

During our junior year of college we moved off campus into an apartment where we finally had a kitchen. We began cooking every night, making a routine where we'd have a scheduled meal for each day of the week. Mondays always seemed to be particularly stressful—long days of chemistry labs packed with pop quizzes and multiple papers due. Monday nights, relieved that the day was over, we'd unwind while we made Monday's comforting open-faced burriot with pumpkin and summer squash. Just the smell of the onions and summer squash stir-frying in the pan immediately calmed us, and as we sat down to eat, we always felt like the weight of the world had been lifted off our shoulders. We now know that there was more to it than our stressful day being over: The summer squash was actually creating a massage from our insides out.

Time to say adios to stress eating and the larger waistline that comes from it. Enter summer squash! One raw cup of this vitamin C powerhouse provides a whopping 32 percent of your daily vitamin C needs. Vitamin C packs a double stress-fighting punch to tackle all stress-related woes. High levels of vitamin C have been shown to reduce levels of stress hormones in the blood, while vitamin C also boosts immunity. This is critical; stress hormones weaken immunity, age the body, make it hard to sleep, and increase body fat—and that's even before the cravings and the overeating caused by the stress hormones do a number on you. Just thinking about the damage these stress hormones creates is anxiety-inducing! It's reassuring to know that vitamin C is hard at work, fighting all of this. What's more, your body requires even more vitamin C when under duress.

Feeling under pressure? There's another reason to munch on some

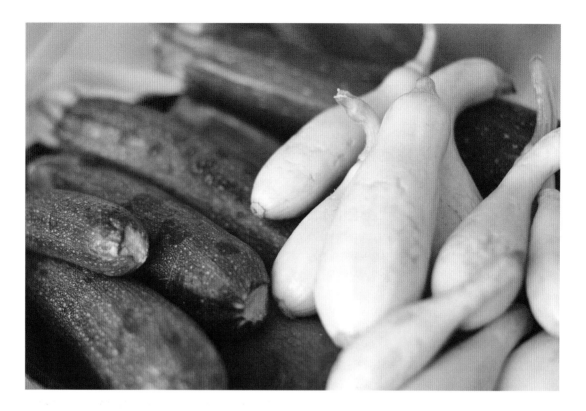

summer squash crudités. Zucchini or yellow squash, it doesn't matter—whichever you choose will help you, since they've both got B vitamins. Your body requires more energy when you're under stress, and B vitamins are essential for your body to create energy. Plus, fall short on them and you're more likely to experience anxiety and depression. B vitamins also are needed for your nervous system and digestive system, so they play a role in how well you respond to stressful situations. Skimp on your summer squash or your B vitamins and you'll be a bundle of nerves.

Folic acid is a specific B vitamin that is crucial during times of stress. If you don't get enough, it can trigger mental fatigue, confusion, forgetfulness, and insomnia. This will only add to your anxiety woes. Got a lot on your plate? Our Vegetable Ribbons are calling your name. Or maybe that's our Zucchini Canoes you hear.

Make sure summer squash is no stranger at your dinner table, and stress will affect you even less. Summer squash is a great source of tension-taming potassium, which is essential for fighting life's hassles. You'll get 8 percent of your daily requirement in a cup of squash. Potassium relaxes your blood vessels and lowers blood pressure. Imagine the blood vessels in your body being squeezed, as if they were wearing a supertight corset. This makes your insides tense as it restricts blood flow. Your entire body feels the pressure. Now imagine potassium swiftly sweeping in and unzipping those tight corsets, relieving the pressure around your vessels. Suddenly you feel free, at ease, your body relaxed. Goodbye, neck kinks caused by stress. Thank you, potassium!

Summer squash doesn't fail us when it comes to magnesium, copper, or omega-3 fatty acids, either. This is important, since magnesium relaxes our muscles and our bodies; copper protects your immune system so you won't succumb to illness at times when your immunity is lowered by stress; omega-3s help reverse tension symptoms by boosting the body's feel-good chemical serotonin and by suppressing the production of adrenaline and cortisol. No time for a bubble bath? Dive into our Rockin' Ratatouille.

There's No Squashing Summer Squash's Health Benefits

Summer squash is a surprisingly powerful source of antioxidant nutrients. Some of these antioxidants are the eye-healthy carotenoids lutein and zeaxanthin. They are bona fide eye protectors—they guard against age-related macular degeneration and cataracts. Additionally, thanks to the B vitamins, folate, choline, zinc, magnesium, fiber, and omega-3 acids that summer squash contains, it helps with healthy blood sugar regulation. Those

very same omega-3 fats and carotenoids exhibit powerful anti-inflammatory and anticancer benefits.

> **Trying to decide whether to steam, boil, or microwave your summer squash? Steam it. You'll retain a good deal more antioxidants—even if you are choosing frozen squash.**

Spotlight on Green Beans

Recipes with Green Beans: Green Bean Salad with Toasted Almonds and Dates, page 218; Quinoa with Mixed Vegetables, page 193; Dieter's Delight Chock Full of Veggies Soup, page 163; Green Beans with Lemon Caper Vinaigrette, page 217

It was a big deal in her house when Tammy's twin girls, Summer and Riley, were able to move on from oatmeal and introduce green vegetables into their diet. Tammy gave a lot of thought to which green veggie she should introduce first. Being a veggie-loving nutritionist, she feared that her daughters would spit out their first bite of vegetables, creating a lifelong mother/daughter veggie struggle. Tammy finally decided that her girls should try green beans first. She thought the green bean's mild, yet delicious, flavor would entice the girls to eat more without turning them off from other veggies in the future. You can only imagine Tammy's delight when after Summer and Riley's first bite of green beans, they squealed for more. And the

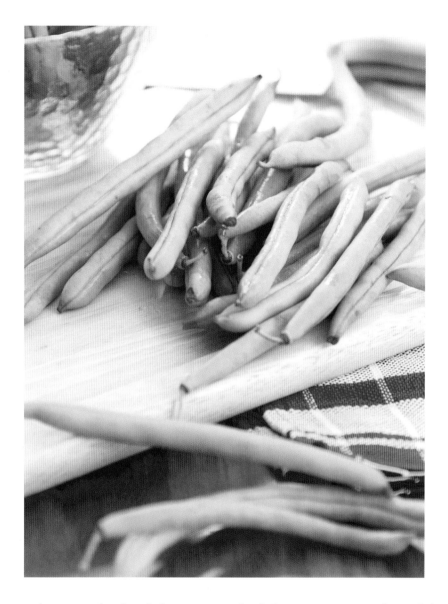

best part was knowing that her babies were getting a lot of nutrients from the green beans, including ones that would help to calm them, even when they were at their fussiest.

Green beans tame tension and tiredness, making them a true champion in the fight against stress. Stressful, tiring day at work? Release your tension in minutes by munching on steamed green beans. Here's why: They help the body to create energy, which we all need more of, especially when under pressure. All of this is thanks to green beans' B vitamins, like folate, B_1, B_2, B_3, and B_6. Under stress, the body experiences a reduction in these vital nutrients, which help the nervous system to fight anxiety and sadness. So it's essential to get even more if you are under the gun.

If you've had a bad day, enjoy a serving of our Green Beans with Lemon Caper Vinaigrette. They'll thwart cravings and stress eating, since they're loaded with vitamin C, which provides potent protection against stress. Research has shown that if you can get enough vitamin C, you may actually be able to stop the flow of stress hormones, which is appealing for several reasons. These stress hormones are the same ones that make your body superefficient at storing body fat, so not only will you avoid stress eating, but you'll store less body fat and be slimmer. And this alone helps to reduce stress! Vitamin C is also a powerful immune-boosting nutrient, which helps to protect cells from the damage that stress causes.

Green beans are a good source of muscle-relaxing magnesium. Magnesium and calcium are depleted quickly and needed in greater quantities when your body is under stress. When magnesium and calcium in the body drop, you'll quickly fall prey to muscle tension and cramps. Tight muscles only increase body tension and exacerbate stress. As calcium drops, you are at risk for a weak body and weak bones.

No time to simply take a breath, let alone to meditate? Enjoy some green beans. Green beans provide both a tryptophan and a potassium boost. Tryptophan increases levels of serotonin, the neurotransmitter and body feel-good chemical and sedative. Potassium is an electrolyte that works with tryptophan, conducting nerve impulses and keeping the brain's neurotransmitters, like serotonin, working properly. Potassium also keeps blood pressure down, minimizing the strain inside your entire body.

It doesn't end there. Green beans provide the body with mood-stabilizing iron, immune-protecting copper, and depression-fighting omega-3s. Green Bean Salad with Toasted Almonds and Dates, anyone?

There's Gold in This Green Bean

Aside from being the next best thing to yoga for fighting stress, green beans contain a combination of calcium and magnesium, making them stellar for bone health. Green beans' powerful antioxidants make them excellent for heart health and the diseases like cancer that they protect against. Carotenoid and flavonoid compounds found in green beans provide defense against cancer, type 2 diabetes, and inflammatory diseases.

The ideal steaming time for green bean nutrient retention and flavor is five minutes.

CHAPTER 2

Beat the Bloat and Clean the Pipes

Veggies for Belly Relief

The Problem: It's a bad day for your abdomen, and you're experiencing bloating, gas, and belly bulges.

Here's What You Need: Vegetables, particularly steamed ones packed with potassium, water, and fiber. If your gut is sensitive when you eat fiber (that is, you experience gas or bloating), choose steamed veggies rather than raw ones, since heating breaks down some of the fiber. This means cooked veggies require your gastrointestinal tract to work less to digest the fiber, and the fiber will pass more quickly through the colon, keeping distention to a minimum. If your colon must work to digest fiber for a long time, there's time for bacteria to ferment and cause bloating.

Here's Why: Let's face it, who doesn't want a flat stomach? To get it, you need foods that will keep your digestive tract moving, so that you can flush out all of the irritants. The last thing you want to eat is heavy or fatty foods, since they take hours to digest and blow you up more. You need food that is light. Often you feel bloated because you have had too much salt. Both potassium and water will help flush excess sodium out of the body. Constipation is another reason you experience belly bloat and bulges. Fiber, aided by the water and potassium in veggies, helps to flush waste out of the body and create a flatter stomach.

Here's How to Get It: For water and potassium, include vegetables like fennel, cucumbers, summer squash, romaine and red leaf lettuce, and tomatoes. For roughage, include leafy greens, artichokes, bell peppers, and mushrooms.

Note: If you often experience constipation and the accompanying bloat, you may have found that cruciferous vegetables like broccoli, cauliflower, cabbage, and brussels sprouts—thanks to their fiber— help to push food out of your colon that's been lingering and causing discomfort. For some people this is the reason steamed and cooked cruciferous veggies are the ultimate bloat-busting prescription. However, others find that although these veggies help to prevent constipation, they create gas and bloating. Based on your body's response, use your judgment to decide if cruciferous veggie recipes should be part of your personal Veggie Cure anti-bloat prescription.

Spotlight on Fennel

Recipes with Fennel: Bengali Cabbage, page 205; Fennel Stuffed Potatoes, page 189; Roasted Fennel, page 231; Rockin' Ratatouille, page 152

Like all good love affairs, ours with fennel began in an Italian restaurant. It was a house salad that had been spruced up by a chopped fennel bulb that had us raving and in disbelief that it was simply a vegetable. Fennel added such a sweet, aromatic crunchiness to the salad. We thought for sure we must be swallowing far more calories than we cared to admit for such a divine flavor. Since then, it's a rare day that you don't see us picking up fennel at our local market.

If you're a fan of licorice like us, you'll automatically enjoy fennel, as its flavor has been described as reminiscent of licorice—but fennel enables you to indulge without all of the calories, added sugar, subsequent crash, or intestinal upset and belly bloat that often accompany sugar-laden foods and candies like licorice.

Have an unsettled tummy? Feeling bloated, constipated, or just that your digestive tract is on the fritz? Fennel is the supreme anti-bloater you should go for. If you've ever needed some stomach settling, someone may have suggested fennel tea or chewing on fennel seeds to ease the problem. Both have been recommended for reducing gas, heartburn,

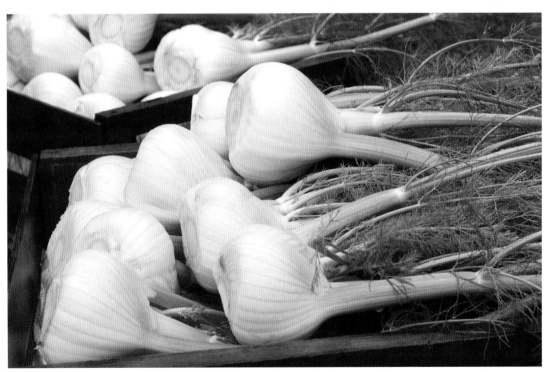

and bloating. In fact, research shows that fennel may be an effective treatment for colic—those digestive woes that seem so difficult to treat and cause some babies to cry at no end.

Feeling a little uncomfortable? No need to admit that you have constipation or the unsightly gut bulges that come with it. Just have some fennel and it will all be history. Consider that in one cup of fennel you'll receive 2.7 grams of fiber (10.8 percent of the daily value)—so it will keep food moving swiftly through your digestive tract. It also will flush out intestinal irritants that may be likely to cause inflammation, bloat, gas, and discomfort. Think of the fiber in fennel like the after-school guard on the playground, who keeps the kids moving off and prevents any stragglers from staying on the grounds, where they could stir up trouble. The fiber prevents any foods or toxins from lingering in the colon where they could lead to digestive issues and bloat.

> Dehydration is another cause for discomfort, constipation, and bloating; fluid is needed to push waste out of the colon. Fennel is 90 percent water, so it helps to hydrate and flush the colon.

A lack of potassium, which helps to regulate fluid in the body, also often causes constipation. A cup of fennel provides 10.3 percent of the DV for potassium. And potassium doesn't just fight the bloat due to constipation—you can also kiss bloating from salt good-bye! That's because potassium counteracts sodium and helps to flush out excess salt along with the surplus of water that comes with salt.

If you didn't already want to dive into our Fennel Stuffed Potatoes, consider that they will provide you with immune-boosting phytonutrients that'll keep digestive organs free of inflammation and disturbance. Although this is good news for your tummy, it's fantastic for your entire body, since keeping your digestive tract healthy is essential to ensuring that the whole body is healthy. If you were to flatten out all of the little folds (villi) of the small intestine, it would cover a football field!

Beyond the Bloat

In the past, fennel has not been seen as having much nutritional value. However, fennel is a powerful immune booster. It has ample vitamin C and molybdenum, and its folic acid makes it great for the heart and for pregnancy. It helps keep energy levels high with niacin. Fennel assists in keeping bones strong with calcium, manganese, and magnesium, and its iron helps to fight anemia. Obviously, fennel's hardly devoid of nutrient value! What's more, fennel helps reduce inflammation, aids in preventing oxidative damage and cancer, and protects the liver from toxic injury. Care for some Roasted Fennel?

For easy digestion, don't underestimate the power of chewing. Since digestive enzymes can only work on the surface of the food fragments, inadequate chewing results in incomplete digestion because food particles are so big. This means not only that nutrients will not get absorbed but that extra food will also be in the colon for bacteria. This results in bacterial overgrowth, gas, and symptoms of indigestion.

Spotlight on Artichokes

Recipes with Artichokes: Artichoke Hummus, page 126; Parmesan Baked Artichoke, page 148; Tomato Artichoke Pasta Bake, page 201

The first time we had a whole artichoke didn't come until we were adults. We had eaten some scrumptious artichoke dips before then (try our delicious low-calorie Artichoke Hummus) but never an entire artichoke. Our first experience was at our favorite Italian restaurant around the corner from where we live on Manhattan's Upper West Side. We had been there countless times and never paid attention to the garlic and wine artichoke that was always featured as an appetizer. It wasn't until artichokes started to get a lot of attention for ranking among the highest in antioxidants that even we noticed it on the menu and tried it for ourselves. Once we tried it, we were hooked! In fact, we enjoyed it so

much that we have been creating our own variations of the dish and other recipes with whole artichokes ever since. And as it turns out, every time we treat ourselves to an artichoke, we also are aiding our digestion and making it a little bit easier to slip on our jeans.

Artichokes are known to ease digestion. Even the ancient Greeks and Romans noticed the benefits and considered artichokes a valuable digestive aid. And nowadays Germany's Commission E, the governmental regulatory agency, has authorized the artichoke leaf for treatment of problems like intestinal discomfort, bloating, lack of appetite, nausea, and mild diarrhea or constipation. The leaf of the artichoke stimulates bile production, which plays a large role in digestion. It's the artichoke's phytochemicals, particularly chlorogenic acid, that are responsible for these benefits. This season's trend forecast: artichokes in, abdominal problems out.

Artichoke ranks among the foods highest in fiber. In fact, one medium artichoke, with a whopping 7 grams of fiber, has more fiber than a cup of prunes! Hello, nature's liquid plumber! That's 28 percent of the amount that you need daily to sweep your colon clean. Without the fiber to push waste along, your intestines can get blocked, causing discomfort and other problems.

Too much Chinese food, salty french fries, or chips? Our Parmesan Baked Artichoke is just the quick remedy you're looking for. Packed with potassium to

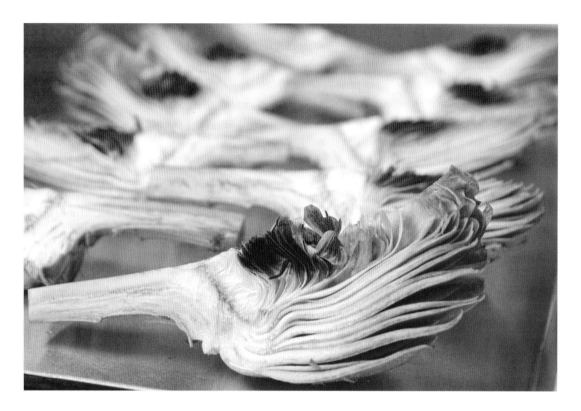

help balance your body's fluid and counteract all of that bloating salt, artichokes help to flush salt out and leave you feeling bloat-free.

More than Just Bloat-Free

In addition to their anti-bloat nutrients (fiber, potassium, and phytonutrients), artichokes are now known for topping the list of the vegetables highest in antioxidants, thanks to the powerful phytonutrients cynarin and silymarin, which have strong positive effects on the liver. Artichokes have been reputed to help in the cure of liver cancer and other liver diseases and to help fight heart disease and diabetes. Artichokes are rich in antioxidants such as vitamin C and are a good source of energy-revving B vitamins like niacin, vitamin B_6, and folic acid. They contain iron, phosphorous, vitamin K, magnesium, copper, and manganese as well to keep your bones and your cells healthy, among other things.

> Canned artichokes contain added salt. If you're trying to cut sodium, rinse the artichokes to reduce the salt.

CHAPTER 3

I Heart My Veggies

Veggies That Keep Your Cardiovascular System in Tune

The Problem: Heart disease is the number one killer in the United States. Did you know that most of the risk factors for heart disease are completely preventable? Unfortunately people often make two wrong choices: They choose unhealthy foods, and they skimp on exercise—or skip it entirely. Fast food, most prepared foods, fatty and processed meats, butter, cream, ice cream, fried foods, biscuits, cookies, candies, and cakes are all a double whammy on the heart. These foods are high in saturated and trans fat, sodium, and sugar and low in fiber and nutrients.

These poor food choices contribute to the risk factors for heart disease, such as high cholesterol and high blood pressure, that can lead to clogged heart vessels and arteries, all of which put a strain on the heart. To make matters worse, these foods trigger the release of harmful stimulants that cause inflammation (swelling) of the arteries. Swollen arteries mean less space for blood to flow, so it's easier for them to become clogged; vessels become ticking time bombs that prevent oxygenated blood from getting to the heart and the rest of the body. The inflammation simultaneously causes the release of damaging free radicals, resulting in a drastic increase in the risk of heart disease, heart attack, stroke, and peripheral arterial disease.

The great news is that by making changes in your lifestyle (we'll focus on what you can do with your diet) you can actually reduce your risk for heart disease.

Heart Disease Risk Factors Directly Affected by Diet:

- High LDL, or "bad" cholesterol

- Low HDL, or "good" cholesterol

- Uncontrolled hypertension (high blood pressure)

- Obesity (more than 20 percent over one's ideal body weight)

- Uncontrolled diabetes

- High C-reactive protein

Other Risk Factors for Heart Disease:

- Physical inactivity

- Smoking

- Uncontrolled stress and anger

Here's What You Need: A heart-healthy eating plan including at least five servings of veggies a day. The keys to your heart-healthy eating plan are:

- **Fruits and vegetables:** at least 4½ cups a day. All types help to keep your ticker healthy, but our specific recommendations are targeted for heart health.

- **Fish:** at least two 3½-ounce servings a week, preferably oily fish like salmon, trout, and herring.

- **Fiber-rich whole grains** like whole wheat, oats, oatmeal, whole rye, whole grain corn, and buckwheat: at least three 1-ounce-equivalent servings a day.

- **Limited sodium:** less than 1,500 milligrams a day. Look for low-sodium and low-fat varieties of cookies, snack chips, breads, cakes, and baked goods.

- **Limited sugar-sweetened beverages:** no more than 450 calories (36 ounces) a week. That's the equivalent of three cans of soda or 6 ounces of fruit drinks a maximum of three days a week.

Other Dietary Measures:
- Eat nuts, legumes, and seeds: five 1-ounce servings a week.

- Use low-fat/nonfat dairy foods, 2–3 servings daily, if you eat dairy.

- Limit processed meats like bacon, sausage, hot dogs, sandwich meat, packaged ham, pepperoni, and salami to no more than two 3-ounce servings a week.

- Limit saturated fat—in butter, cream, full-fat cheese and milk, palm oil, and palm kernel oil—to less than 7 percent of total energy intake. Try small portions of oils for cooking or baking or in dressings or spreads. Choose options that are the lowest in saturated fat, trans fat, and cholesterol, such as canola oil, corn oil, olive oil, safflower oil, sesame oil, soybean oil, and sunflower oil.

- Stay away from palm oil, palm kernel oil, coconut oil, and cocoa butter. Even though they are vegetable oils and have no cholesterol, they're high in saturated fats. Although coconut oil does have some encouraging health research, it is premature to recommend it.

- Choose reduced-fat, low-fat, light, or fat-free salad dressings (if you need to limit your calories) to use with salads, for dips, or as marinades.

- Avoid trans fat by rejecting margarines that don't specify 0 grams of trans fat, as well as any product with "partially hydrogenated" ingredients.

The best way to combat heart disease is to squash the risk factors. This means attacking heart disease before it becomes a reality, by avoiding foods that increase cholesterol levels, inflammation, blood pressure, and the risk of obesity. Instead, choose foods that increase the body's immunity and raise the body's good cholesterol. Although every vegetable can play a part in improving heart health, some vegetables are more beneficial than others. Choosing the best I Heart My Veggies and eating them with this heart-healthy eating plan can take your heart health to a whole new level. You can attack heart disease before it has the chance to get at you.

Think of your arteries and veins as a giant tunnel system: the more smooth, pliable, and free of clogs, damage, and leaks the tunnels are, the more efficient the system. Keeping the tunnels smooth and like new helps to prevent heart disease. Your ultimate weapons in the prevention of heart disease are the vegetables highest in potassium, B vitamins, antioxidants, and soluble fiber. The combination of these nutrients in high amounts explains why black beans, crimini mushrooms, garlic, and Swiss chard are I Heart My Veggies extraordinaires.

Here's Why:

• **Potassium counterbalances sodium.** This makes potassium a major player in the prevention of heart disease. Salt is also a major culprit in clogging the pipes. Since excess salt intake leads to excess water in the blood, there is more pressure in your blood vessels, and

your heart has to work harder. This is what we call high blood pressure, or hypertension. Potassium fights the damage sodium does by helping to reduce the risk of high blood pressure. Sodium also increases inflammation, making your blood vessels stiff, and this too makes it harder for blood to pump. Since potassium helps flush out sodium, it also protects the heart by helping keep vessels more elastic and pliable.

Potassium—Where to Find It

Excellent sources of potassium: chard, crimini mushrooms, and spinach

Very good sources of potassium: fennel, mustard greens, brussels sprouts, broccoli, winter squash, blackstrap molasses, eggplant, bell peppers, potatoes, tomatoes, summer squash, celery, romaine lettuce, cauliflower, turnip greens, asparagus, shiitake mushrooms, kale, carrots, beets, and green beans

Good sources of potassium: cucumbers, avocados, sweet potatoes and cabbage

Note: Low-fat dairy foods help lower blood pressure and are packed with potassium; when eaten in combination with veggies and a low-sodium diet, they help to protect the heart. That's why they'll be included in recipes linked to this chapter.

• **Antioxidants protect the heart.**
The health of our circulatory system
depends on antioxidant protection
and on keeping inflammation at bay.
Antioxidant and anti-inflammatory
nutrients can help protect us from
cardiovascular disease by protecting our
blood vessels from oxidative damage and
chronic inflammation.

• **Each of the I Heart My Veggies offers
specific phytonutrients,** each with
different cardiovascular benefits. *Phyto-*
means "plant," and phytonutrients
(a.k.a. phytochemicals) come from
plants. Phytonutrients are a relatively
recent discovery in the nutrition world,
and they are turning out to be really
important. It's been well accepted for
many years that people who eat a lot of
vegetables and fruits are healthier in
many ways. It was believed that this was
due to the rich amounts of vitamins
and minerals in vegetables and fruits.
But it turns out that in addition to
the vitamins and minerals, there
are thousands of other substances,
phytonutrients, that are beneficial to
humans. In plants, they seem to help
form a protective shield against the
environment, including preventing
disease. Phytonutrients seem to protect
us in similar ways. They can repair
damage to cells, help build our immune
systems, and act as antioxidants. Of
course, this means they help protect the
cardiovascular system, which explains
why we "heart" our phytonutrients.

As kids, our favorite colors were
bright and colorful shades of turquoise,
green, and pink, so it's no surprise that
our love affair with color continues. We
adore phytochemicals for what they do
to keep us healthy, but also because they
are actually responsible for producing
the bright colors in fruits and veggies.
The purple cabbage, the green spinach,
the red bell pepper, and the blueberry
can all credit their gorgeous hues to
their phytochemicals.

Because bright colors produced
by phytochemicals signal health benefits, this is where the saying "Eat your
colors" or "Eat the rainbow of colors"
comes from. It's also significant that
each of these foods contains many different phytochemicals that can tackle
different damaging oxidation reactions in our cells. Therefore each phytochemical and each vegetable has a
slightly different effect in our bodies.
This is why it is important to eat a variety of fruits and vegetables. This means
don't forget about the less popular
parsnips and turnips. Go for our I Beg
Your Parsnips (page 146) and you'll get
a "heart"-y dose of soluble fiber, potassium, and folic acid.

• **B vitamins (like vitamin B_6 and
folate) help lower homocysteine,** an
amino acid in the blood. Homocysteine
may promote atherosclerosis (fatty
deposits in blood vessels) by damaging
the inner lining of arteries and
promoting blood clots. Although a

causal link hasn't been established, people at high risk for heart disease should be sure to get enough folic acid and vitamins B_6 and B_{12} in their diet, since these nutrients may be protective for other reasons. They should eat fruits and green, leafy vegetables daily.

> Research has shown that increasing soluble fiber by 5 to 10 grams a day reduces LDL cholesterol by about 5 percent. Go for our I Beg Your Parsnips, (page 146) and you'll get a "heart"-y dose (3 grams!) plus B_6, folate, and potassium. Oat bran and oatmeal, as well as psyllium and barley, are rich in beta-glucan, a soluble form of fiber, which has been shown to lower total cholesterol and LDL cholesterol. Try our Tomato, Spinach, Egg 'n' Feta Never Tasted Betta Wrap (page 123)—it's made with spinach and oat bran pita.

• **Fiber lowers cholesterol levels.**
Fiber is the part of the plant that is not broken down in the intestines by human digestive enzymes. Since it's not digested, it's not absorbed. Although soluble fiber is more effective at lowering cholesterol, both soluble fiber and insoluble fiber are good for your health, and most vegetables contain some of each. While there is not a large list of vegetables that are high in soluble fiber, broccoli, brussels sprouts, celery, carrots, cucumbers, beans, dried peas, artichokes, parsnips, sweet potatoes,

and turnips are all good for your heart and your digestive system. Soluble fiber is responsible for pulling "bad" LDL cholesterol out of the body.

Here's How to Get It: Eat potatoes, spinach, acorn squash, avocados, and mushrooms for potassium; bell peppers, spinach, baked potatoes (skin included), green peas, yams, broccoli, asparagus, and turnip greens for vitamin B_6; dark leafy greens, asparagus, broccoli, beans, peas, avocados, brussels sprouts, cauliflower, and beets for folic acid. Almost all vegetables are good sources of phytonutrients and fiber.

Although we love all muscles, if we had to choose one, the heart would be our favorite. If the heart stops beating, we can kiss all of our veggies good-bye! So the veggies that play the largest part in keeping the heart healthy are some of the most powerful and important to include in your regular vegetable intake.

Spotlight on Black Beans

Recipes with Black Beans: Corn and Bean Salsa, page 131; Hot Diggity Chili!, page 195; Ole! Mexican Cabbage with Black Beans and Avocados, page 179; Veggie Yard Dash Salad, page 183

Even as kids, we learned that beans are good for the heart. In fact, we have early memories of singing the famous song as we'd devour one of our all-time favorite meals, a taco salad with black beans. And black beans are even more exceptional than the typical bean. Just one cup of black beans provides more than 4 grams of cholesterol-lowering soluble fiber. And research shows that higher intake of soluble fiber is linked with lower risk of coronary heart disease (CHD) and heart attack.

Although you may think of brightly colored fruits and veggies as the best sources of phytochemicals and antioxidants, black beans are actually one of the best sources of the flavonoid compound anthocyanins, typically known for being abundant in red, purple, and blue produce such as red grapes, purple cabbage, raspberries, and cranberries. The outermost layer responsible for the color of the bean is an incredible source of three anthocyanin flavonoids: delphinidin, petunidin, and malvidin.

There are a number of other powerful flavonoids in black beans that are difficult to pronounce and spell, let alone memorize. So don't worry about knowing their names; the most important thing to know is that these potent phytonutrients act as antioxidants *and*

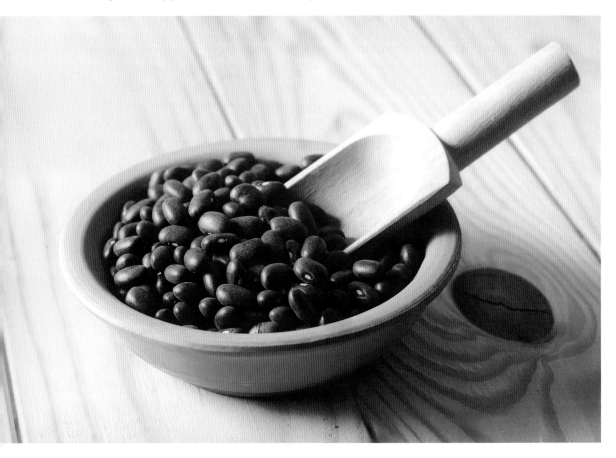

as anti-inflammatory compounds, and both are critical for overall cardiovascular health. When our blood vessels are exposed to chronic and high levels of oxidative stress (damage) or inflammation, they are at an increased risk for disease development. Since black beans are such a stellar food, fabulous at lessening both of these threats, they squash damage that would normally promote disease and thereby decrease the risk of most cardiovascular diseases. Thank you, anthocyanins and other flavonoids in black beans!

Already the case for I Heart My Black Beans is made. However, if you need more convincing, imagine this . . . What if every time you felt uptight or stressed out, your body got a massage from the inside that could result in your muscles and your blood vessels relaxing and therefore improving blood flow, reducing the risk of irregular heart rhythms or spasms of the heart muscle or a blood vessel?

Well, imagine no more. One cup of black beans provides about 120 milligrams of magnesium, close to one-third of the daily value, making them a masseuse for your insides. They are a good source of folate, which seems to be an important B vitamin for decreasing cardiovascular disease risk, and contain antioxidant minerals like zinc and manganese. All of these factors help keep your love muscle in good working order! Black beans and rice, Corn and Bean Salsa, or Black Beans and Avocado, anyone?

Note: Black beans are exceptional when it comes to extending an energy boost. They're also digestive tract supporters (which is a surprise to most people) and diabetes fighters. Animal and laboratory studies are quite consistent in their findings, and studies have shown that black beans inhibit the development of certain cancers, especially colon cancer.

Spotlight on Crimini (a.k.a. Baby Bella) Mushrooms

Recipes with Criminis: Baby Bellas and Asparagus, page 206; Heavenly Roasted Vegetables, page 219; Hickory Broccoli Salad, page 175; Mediterranean Pizza, page 192; Rockin' Ratatouille, page 152; Veggie Frittata Bites, page 121; Sweet and Savory Pumpkin Quiche, page 120

See chapter 12 under "Spotlight on Portobello Mushrooms" (page 73) to see how our love affair with the mature version of crimini mushrooms began. Other than the fact that our Roasted Red Pepper, Spinach, and Feta Portobello Burger (page 196) will make your heart skip a beat, crimini mushrooms (like all mushrooms) provide the satisfying mouth feel of actual meat. However, rather than raising your risk for heart disease as many red meats do, crimini mushrooms do the opposite.

Crimini mushrooms, sometimes called brown mushrooms, are a tan or light brown variety like the button mushroom. White button, crimini, and

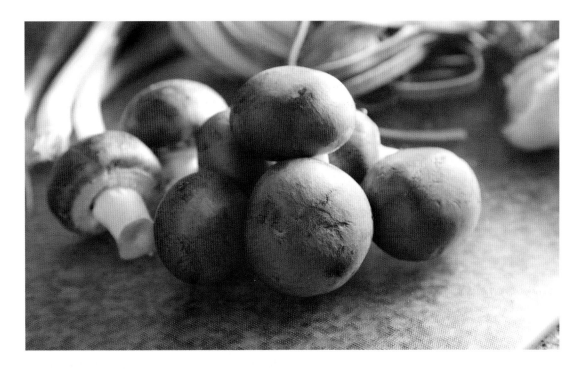

portobello are all the same scientific category of mushroom, *Agaricus bisporus*. White button varieties are usually taken from select strains that can be harvested at a relatively immature stage of growth. Strains used to produce crimini mushrooms are typically harvested at an intermediate growth stage. Baby bella, mini bella, baby portobello, and portobellini are other names for crimini mushrooms. Portobello mushrooms are crimini mushrooms that have been allowed to grow to full maturity.

Crimini mushrooms are packed with heart-healthy potassium, and they contain powerful antioxidant and anti-inflammatory nutrients that protect the heart from oxidative damage and chronic inflammation. They particularly help to combat the risk of cardiovascular disease by protecting the lining of the aorta and by reducing the risk of blood flow problems. Have high cholesterol and want an easy way to reduce your levels of all three blood fats (total cholesterol, LDL cholesterol, and triglycerides) and reduce your risk of heart disease even more? Eat crimini mushrooms daily over a one- to two-month period.

Crimini mushrooms also are an excellent source of B vitamins, so they help keep homocysteine levels in check to keep the heart healthy.

There are two keys to reaping the heart benefits of mushrooms. First, store mushrooms properly so they don't lose their powerful phytonutrients. Discoloration is a sign that your mushrooms won't contain the same powerful heart-protecting properties that they once did. Keep your mushrooms refrigerated: an ideal temperature is 38°F (3°C). When you come home from the grocery store, immediately put them in the refrigerator and avoid leaving them on the counter or storing them in a cabinet.

The second key: Don't overcook your mushrooms. Ideally, sauté them for about seven minutes. Your heart will thank you.

Note: Crimini mushrooms (like porto-bellos and white button) offer exceptional benefits when it comes to warding off cancer, keeping skin youthful, reliev-ing stress, and boosting mood.

Spotlight on Swiss Chard

Recipes with Swiss Chard: Swiss Chard Salad with Red and Golden Beets and Honey Yogurt Vinaigrette, page 182; Simple Sautéed Spinach, page 234

If you are like us and most of our clients, then you didn't grow up with Swiss chard (also called chard) on your dinner plate. But after trying some braised chard at a trendy restaurant (for us it was in New York City's meatpacking district) or after learning just how important it is to add leafy greens to your diet, you'll won-der why you haven't eaten it more often. After all, Swiss chard belongs to the same family as beets and spinach, and its bitter, pungent, and slightly salty flavor will make you feel like you just can't get enough of our I Heart My Swiss Chard recipes.

Remember that one of the key fac-tors of heart health is preventing oxida-tive stress. Sure, chard's an excellent source of the traditional antioxidants that do this (vitamin C, vitamin E, beta-carotene) and a good source of the minerals manganese and zinc that help scavenge free radicals and prevent oxida-tive damage. But what keeps our hearts aflutter is that recent research shows that chard leaves contain an array of polyphe-nol antioxidants, including kaempferol, the heart-protective flavonoid that's also found in broccoli, kale, strawberries, and other foods.

The phytonutrient antioxidants in chard that play a part in protecting the cardiovascular system include carot-enoids (beta-carotene, lutein, and zea-xanthin, which lend plants their green and orange hues), flavonoids (quercetin, red hues) and kaempferol (white and creamy hues). This broad range of phy-tonutrients in chard is even more exten-sive than researchers initially suspected: Three dozen antioxidant phytonutrients have been identified in chard! So if you want to fight cardiovascular disease, eat-ing chard is one of the best things you can do to keep your heart in good work-ing order. Many of these antioxidant phytonutrients provide chard with its colorful stems, stalks, and leaf veins.

And if our hearts weren't already beating a bit faster, an additional bonus is that many of the incredible

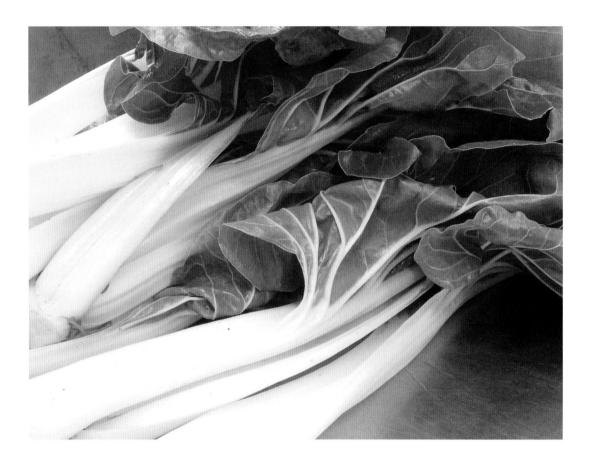

phytonutrient antioxidants in chard also act as anti-inflammatory agents. These beneficial phytonutrients sometimes lower the risk of chronic inflammation by interfering with the action of enzymes that cause it. At other times they intercede at the very first step of inflammation. Since chronic low-level inflammation, especially when coupled with excessive oxidative stress, increases our risk of atherosclerosis and high blood pressure, chard is a key vegetable for lowering the risk of these health problems.

Add to these benefits that chard is an excellent source of heart-healthy potassium, folate, and fiber, and you've got yourself one "Heart"-y veggie! Braised chard, anyone?

Ensuring Knock-out Nutrients

For the best-tasting chard and to make sure that the nutrients are retained, choose a bunch that is kept in a chilled display. This will also ensure a crunchier texture and sweeter taste. Look for vivid green leaves that aren't browning or yellowing. The leaves should not be wilted and shouldn't have tiny holes. The stalks should look crisp and be unblemished.

Note: Chard is one of only three vegetables that we recommend boiling to help reduce its concentration of oxalic acid. Oxalic acid binds to the calcium in the chard and makes it hard to absorb. Slice leaves in 1-inch strips and the stems in ½-inch sections and boil for just 3 minutes. Although colored stems on chard look pretty, we only recommend eating the stems of varieties with white stems; colored stems are very tough.

Additional Exceptional Swiss Chard Superpowers:
Blood sugar control, detox support, and bone health

Spotlight on Garlic

Recipes with Garlic (although this book contains a whopping 42 recipes that contain garlic, here we name a handful of our favorites that just wouldn't be the same without it): Artichoke Hummus, page 126; Cauliflower Crusted Mozzarella Pie, page 186; Cold Cucumber and Avocado Soup, page 160; Cream of Whatever Soup, page 159; Eggplant Parmesan, page 187; Golden Gazpacho in Petite Cucumber Cradles, page 139; Jicama Fried Rice, page 226; Just Call Me Baby Bok Choy, page 228; Mediterranean Pizza, page 192; Roasted Garlic Broccolini, page 232; Roasted Tomato Puttanesca, page 199; Spaghetti Squash with Fresh Tomato Sauce, page 200; Tomato and Basil Bruschetta, page 157; Tomato Artichoke Pasta Bake, page 201; The Nutrition Twins' Skinny Cauliflower Mash, page 238

Take a stroll in front of any Italian restaurant and you'll likely be enticed by the wonderfully fragrant scent of garlic. If your mouth waters just at the thought of this, you're not alone. Our clients often tell us that the same is true for them, just as it is for us. The compounds responsible for garlic's recognizable pungent odor are a variety of powerful sulfur-containing compounds called thiosulfinates, sulfoxides, and dithiins. They're also the source of many of garlic's heart benefits, and they're certainly worth making a stink over. Although these compounds are found in other members of the lily or allium family, which includes onions and leeks, garlic is king when it comes to keeping your heart healthy.

What makes garlic so good for the heart? Not only can garlic lower blood triglycerides and total cholesterol by 5 to 15 percent, but garlic's biggest asset is its unique set of sulfur-containing compounds that protect blood cells and vessels from inflammatory and oxidative stress.

Like chard, garlic heads to the root of the problem, working to prevent the activity of molecules that cause inflammation. Ajoene, a sulfur-containing compound in garlic, helps prevent clots from forming inside our blood vessels by keeping blood platelets from becoming too sticky. Hallelujah, garlic!

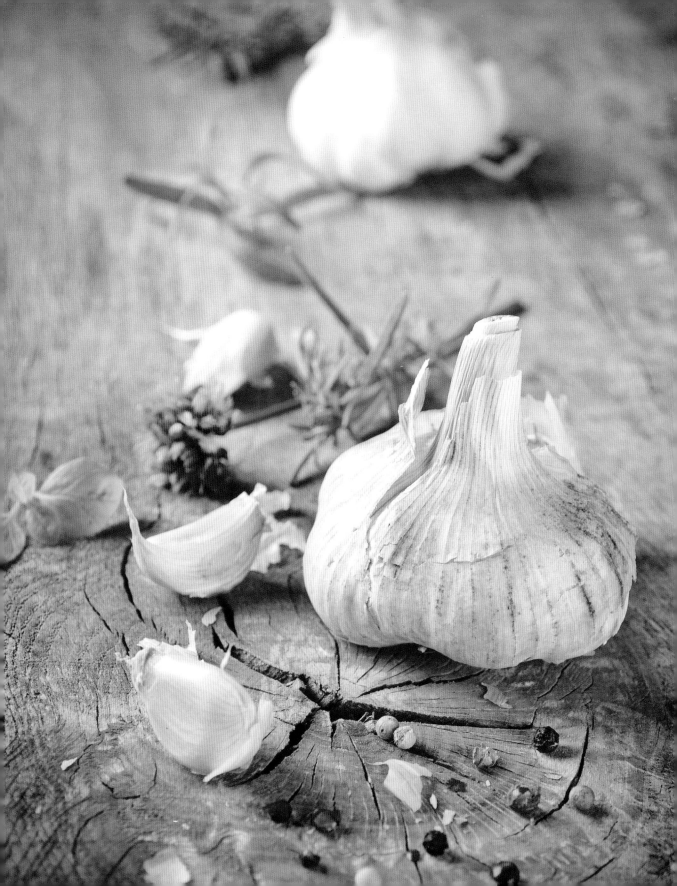

Just in case garlic didn't already have your heart singing, this veggie also lowers blood pressure. Allicin in garlic blocks the activity of angiotensin II, which makes blood vessels contract. When vessels contract, blood is forced to pass through a smaller space, and the pressure is increased. Think of holding a ball of clay in your fist. When you squeeze your hand, the clay gets mushed. By blocking the activity of angiotensin II, allicin in garlic is able to help prevent unwanted contraction of our blood vessels and unwanted increases in blood pressure.

Garlic also supports healthy blood pressure in a second and completely different way. Garlic is rich in sulfur-containing molecules, and our red blood cells use some of these to dilate our blood vessels and to keep our blood pressure in line.

Added bonuses: The vitamin C in garlic protects the heart from damage by shielding LDL cholesterol from oxidation. Since it is the oxidized form of LDL cholesterol that initiates damage to blood vessel walls, a reduction in the levels of oxidizing free radicals in the bloodstream can have a profound effect on preventing cardiovascular disease. Garlic also contains the powerful antioxidants selenium and manganese as well as vitamin B_6, which help lower homocysteine, associated with damage to cell walls.

Note: Although much of the research has been conducted on garlic in supplement form, we will be referring to garlic's benefits in food form, because we agree with the father of modern medicine, Hippocrates, and his famous quote "Let food be thy medicine."

Get the most nutritional bang from your garlic by chopping it or crushing it and letting it sit for five minutes before cooking it or mixing it with other ingredients. Chopping or crushing helps to convert garlic's phytonutrient alliin to the health superstar allicin. Waiting five minutes to cook the chopped garlic and not combining it with lemon or other acidic ingredients will allow for maximal allicin production. Skip this "five-minute wait" and you'll miss out on most of the health benefits.

Garlic has additional superpowers and contributes to the benefits of veggies noted in other chapters including "Stress Relieving and Tension Taming," "Crunching against Cancer," "The Slim & Trim Factor," "Skin Dulgence," and "Mood-Boosting Must-Haves."

CHAPTER 4

Crunching against Cancer

Veggies That Help Reduce Risk

The Problem: One in four deaths in the United States is due to cancer. You realize there are risk factors for cancer that you can't control, but you'd like to do what you can to prevent it by modifying your diet.

Here's What You Need: All veggies. The more the merrier, since they all contain a mix of phytonutrients that have anticancer properties. Be sure to include some of the best veggies for reducing free radicals and those that detoxify carcinogens. Don't know where to begin? Think cruciferous vegetables, like brussels sprouts, arugula, bok choy, broccoli, cabbage, cauliflower, kale, radishes, and turnips. You can also start with veggies in the allium family like onions, garlic, leeks, and chives that can add a lot of flavor to bland meals.

Here's Why: All veggies contain antioxidants that help protect the cells against damage and cancer. Glucosinolates are sulfur-containing compounds found in cruciferous vegetables that stimulate enzymes in the body that detoxify carcinonogens, reduce free radicals, and protect cells from DNA damage. Eat enough veggies—some in particular—and you are doing one of the best things you can do to protect your body against cancer.

Spotlight on Onions

A Few of Our Fave Onion Recipes (24 of our recipes have onions or scallions!): Beet and Carrot Savory Pancakes, page 114; Coco Sweet Potatoes with Mango Salsa, page 130; Potato Bites, page 230; Roasted Tomato Puttanesca, page 199; Sweet and Savory Pumpkin Quiche, page 120; Teriyaki-Lime Veggie and Pineapple Kebabs, page 237; Zucchini Canoes, page 158

Our mom cooked dinner for us every night while we were growing up, and one of the main ingredients she used to flavor her meals was onions. We have fond memories of walking into our kitchen only to find Mom crying while chopping onions. We'd playfully tease her, asking if she was watching *Bambi*, a movie that had produced tears for her as a child. Now, whenever chopping an onion brings either of us to tears, we always think of "Mom and Bambi."

Ironically, the very reason that many people don't enjoy cutting up onions—from the tears it brings to their eyes and, for some, the pungent smell—is the

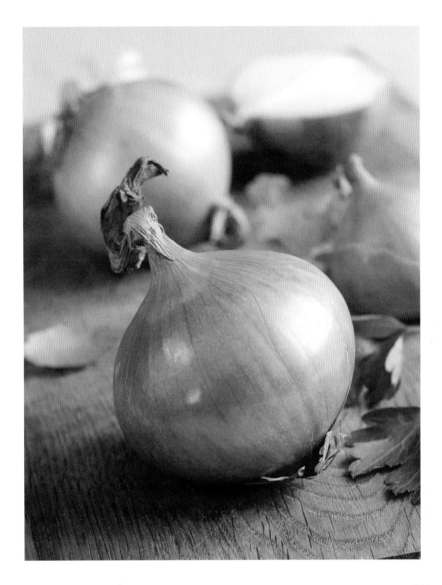

same reason it's beneficial to eat them! The odor-causing sulfur compounds in onions offer numerous benefits.

Do you live on a busy street or near a busy road and breathe in a little soot from the street? Do you spend time with someone who smokes? Do you smell the diesel fumes when you drive on the highway or visit a gas station? Do you use everyday household agents like cleaning solvents, nail polish, or hair spray? Onions help to undo the damage of these cancer-causing environmental toxins. Suddenly the sulfur from the onions doesn't smell so bad. In fact, onions' sulfides also protect against tumor growth.

And research has found that women whose diets are rich in onions have a 40 percent reduction in the risk of ovarian cancer. These sulfides can also explain why studies in Greece have shown that high consumption of onions (and garlic) protects against stomach cancer.

It's not just the sulfur compounds in onions that make them powerful cancer fighters. They are also rich in antioxidants like vitamin C, and in phenolic and flavonoid phytochemicals that squash free radicals by not allowing the substances that damage cells to be produced. In fact, flavonoid consumption has been associated with a reduced risk of cancer (as well as heart disease and diabetes), and onions are the largest source of flavonoids in the human diet.

The key to reaping the benefits is not to "over-peel" the onion, since the outside layers of the flesh tend to be where the flavonoids are most concentrated. So, for the most anticancer benefits, when you take off the onion's outermost layer, peel off as small an amount of the fleshy edible portion as possible. You could lose 20 to 75 percent of the great nutrients if you peel off this valuable cancer-fighting layer. Yes, a slice of onion is certainly worth an ounce of prevention.

A Look beneath the Peel

Besides helping to fight cancer with flavonoids and phenolic and sulfur compounds, onions are rich in the traditional nutrients. Onions are very rich in chromium, a mineral that helps cells respond to insulin, fight diabetes, and regulate blood sugar, and in immune-boosting vitamin C. They are a good source of fiber, bone-healthy manganese, energy-boosting vitamin B_6, and heart-healthy folate and potassium. Onions also have strong anti-inflammatory properties.

How much onion should you eat to reduce your risk of cancer? For ovarian, colorectal, and laryngeal cancer, research shows that one to seven half-cup servings a week seem to be sufficient. Aim for the higher range to play it safe. However, for oral and esophageal cancer, it looks like you need more—one onion serving (roughly half a cup) daily.

The more phenolic and flavonoid antioxidants an onion has, the stronger its ability to fight off cancer. One study found that yellow onions have much stronger anticancer ability than western white onions because they have eleven times more flavonoids.

After cutting onions, let them sit for at least five minutes before cooking them or eating them, to help enhance their health-promoting benefits. The chopping or dicing will rupture the onions' cells and release the cancer-fighting phytonutrient allicin. Allicin gives onions their strong smell and makes your eyes tear. The more your eyes tear and the stronger the smell while you're slicing the onion, the more it will benefit your health!

Spotlight on Brussels Sprouts

Recipes with Brussels Sprouts: Butternut and Turnip Barley Risotto, page 185; Oh Baby! Brussels Sprouts, page 229; Savory Brussels Sprouts, page 233; Stuffed Peppers, page 202

When we were eight years old, we came home from school to find Mom in bed with the flu, sick for the first time. We wanted to comfort her, so we told her to relax, we'd make dinner. Despite its being our first time making dinner, we were determined to get Mom healthy, and we knew just what to make to aid her recovery: Split Pea and Barley Soup (see page 166) to warm her bones (she had taught us that there's nothing better than soup to feel good) and steamed brussels sprouts, since they were one of Mom's favorite veggies and she always told us how good they were for us. We worked for quite some time on dinner, eventually burning the soup, making it inedible, and then overcooking the brussels sprouts. But Mom was a sport and still ate the brussels sprouts and said they were delicious. Lo and behold, the next day Mom was out of bed and feeling much better. To this day, we credit the brussels sprouts.

As usual, Mom was right. Brussels sprouts are good for us; in fact, they're one of the most potent cancer fighters out there. Scores of studies prove that brussels sprouts are powerhouses when it comes to fighting cancer. They not only help prevent cancer, but if you have cancer,

they help you to beat it. That's because they play a major role in three body systems that are involved with cancer—the body's antioxidant system, the body's detox system, and the inflammatory/anti-inflammatory system. When these systems are imbalanced, they increase the risk of cancer. The risk is especially increased when all three systems have imbalances simultaneously. And brussels sprouts provide special nutrient support for all three of these systems. So dive into our Stuffed Peppers that are bursting with brussels sprouts for your daily dose of cancer prevention.

Going to a barbecue? Enjoy some grilled brussels sprouts with your meat and you can fight cancer from many different angles! Grilling and charbroiling meats at high temperatures creates carcinogens (cancer-causing agents) called heterocyclic amines. Brussels sprouts protect against these heterocyclic amines, which are especially associated with colon cancer. In fact, thanks to brussels sprouts' fiber (4 grams a cup!), which nourishes the cell lining of the colon walls, when it comes to detoxifying the body and clearing out the colon, they can reduce precancerous cells in the colon by more than 50 percent. Additionally, those brussels sprouts can reduce precancerous cells in the liver by as much as 70 percent and shrink precancerous cancer lesions by 85 to 91 percent.

It doesn't end at colon and liver cancer. If you want to do all that you can to avoid breast cancer, or if you feel that

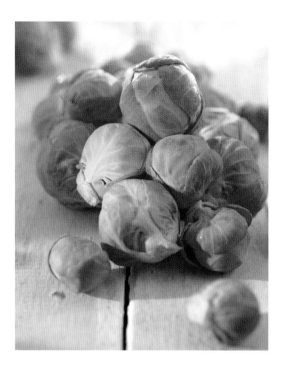

Too busy to fight cancer today? Not with our easy-to-prepare Oh Baby! Brussels Sprouts, you're not! Brussels sprouts' isothiocyanates' potent cancer-fighting properties will help combat bladder cancer. The isothiocyanates travel through the bladder to be excreted and likely work some of their magic as they're passing through. Research has shown that those with the highest intake of brussels sprouts and cruciferous vegetables have a 29 percent lower risk of cancer of the bladder than those who ate the least.

Are you a smoker? Although no amount of vegetables, or anything else for that matter, can undo the damage of smoking, load up on your brussels sprouts. They're especially known for fighting lung cancer as well as ovarian cancer.

your environmental and genetic factors put you at risk for breast cancer, or even if you have breast cancer, now's the time to try our Savory Brussels Sprouts. The sulforaphane found in brussels sprouts helps detoxify cancer-causing chemicals from everything from household products to dry cleaning chemicals. Brussels sprouts are so powerful that they can halt the proliferation of breast cancer cells, even in the late stages of cancer growth.

If you're concerned about yourself or your loved one developing prostate cancer, get three or more servings of cruciferous vegetables like brussels sprouts each week and you can slash the risk of prostate cancer by 44 percent. Not bad, especially when you can enjoy every last bite.

Health Benefits Sprouting Everywhere

Brussels sprouts protect against heart disease with their folate, and they help lower cholesterol thanks to their fiber. Their vitamin K, omega-3 fatty acid, and glucosinolate content makes brussels sprouts a potent anti-inflammatory, helping to battle against some of the damage caused by lack of sleep or exercise, chronic stress, or a poor diet. Their fiber makes them great for digestive health, and so does their glucoraphanin, which helps to keep your insides healthy by preventing bacterial overgrowth.

CHAPTER 5

Bone Boosting Bonanzas

Veggie Recipes Built to Build Strong Bones

The Problem: If you want to be your strongest, healthiest, and sexiest self, a weak skeleton that prevents you from standing up straight isn't going to get you there. While everybody's bones get weaker as we grow older, the effects of aging can be particularly problematic if you already have weak bones or if osteoporosis runs in your family. If you're like most people, you fall short in getting the nutrients that you need to keep your bones healthy.

Think you're too young and sexy for osteoporosis? Not so fast. Bones can be brittle at any age. A University of Arkansas study revealed that 2 percent of college-age women already have osteoporosis. A further 15 percent have sustained significant losses in bone density, and may be well on their way to developing osteoporosis. Often people don't even know they have fragile bones until a bone breaks—and it can happen simply from sneezing, bending forward, or stepping. A broken bone can seriously disrupt your everyday life. A serious injury can cause pain, disability, or loss of independence. Daily activities such as walking without help can become difficult.

Did you know that your bones are actually living, growing tissue? You constantly lose old bone while you make new bone. As children and teenagers, we make bone faster than we lose it, and our bones get denser until we reach our peak bone mass around thirty. Then we gradually lose bone. When we lose too much bone, make too little bone, or both, osteoporosis happens. By maximizing your peak bone mass before the age of thirty, you are less likely to break a bone or get osteoporosis later in life.

Bone loss typically accelerates in both men and women in mid-life. Bone loss usually increases when bone-protective estrogen levels drop after menopause in women, particularly in the five to seven years after menopause, when women can lose up to 20 percent or more of their bone density. But it's never too late at any age to take steps to protect your bones.

When the bones in the spine get weak and break, the breaks cause a person to get shorter. When you see a person with stooped shoulders (a "hunchback"), this is usually the reason why. Certain choices and habits accelerate the process of weakening of the bones, including:

• not getting enough calcium, vitamin D, and other nutrients (we'll focus on helping you to get these nutrients from food rather than vitamin supplements)

- getting too much salt, caffeine, protein

- smoking

- drinking too much alcohol, coffee, and soft drinks

- using certain medications, such as corticosteroids and anticonvulsants

- not engaging in enough weight-bearing exercise, like strength training or walking or running at least 30 minutes on most days

Here's What You Need: A bona fide bone-strengthening meal plan including nutrients that encourage bone strength and prevent bone loss—calcium, vitamin D, vitamin K, magnesium, potassium, and prebiotic fiber from food sources. Plus, researchers have recently found an important connection between lycopene, its antioxidant properties, and bone health. A study found that when you remove lycopene-containing foods like tomatoes from the diet, women are at increased risk of osteoporosis.

Here's Why: No bones about it, one of the sexiest parts of the body is a strong skeleton. A sturdy frame will help you to stand up straight. Good posture exudes confidence—now, that's sexy. With a weak structure, you are like a temple with no pillars.

Calcium, vitamin D, and vitamin K work together to build and repair your bones. Prebiotic fiber, vitamin D, and vitamin K help calcium to be absorbed. Magnesium helps to direct calcium to the bones. Potassium helps to prevent calcium salts from being released from the bones. Calcium salts leave the bones when you ingest too much salt, protein, and cola, which all make the blood too acidic. The calcium salts make the blood more alkaline, but by leaving the bones, they weaken them.

Here's How to Get It: A milk mustache isn't the only way to get calcium for building strong bones. Add these nutrients to your diet and you'll be well on your way to that mighty, attractive skeleton.

- **Go for dark leafy greens** like collard greens, turnip greens, kale, spinach, bok choy (Chinese cabbage), dandelion greens, mustard greens, parsley, watercress, and broccoli. In calcium content, 4 cups of cooked broccoli equal a cup of milk. Try kidney beans, navy beans, black beans, and soy beans and their products like tofu.

  Your body doesn't absorb calcium well from foods that are high in oxalates (derivatives of oxalic acid) such as spinach. Other high-oxalate foods are rhubarb, Swiss chard, and beet greens. These foods contain other healthy nutrients; they just shouldn't be counted as sources of calcium unless you choose to eat them after having boiled them, which unbinds the oxalates. In general, we recommend that you don't boil your vegetables, as you lose a lot of nutrients (water-soluble vitamins are lost in the boiling water). However, in the case of spinach, beet greens, and Swiss chard, boiling them is an acceptable way to prepare them, as it releases more than 50 percent of the oxalates.

• **For a "bad-to-the-bone" skeleton, you need vitamin K.** Think of vitamin K as the glue that binds calcium to the bone. It's necessary for making a protein called osteocalcin, which is needed to bind calcium to the bone matrix, cutting down on calcium excretion in the urine. If you don't get enough of it, osteocalcin will be low, reducing bone mineral density. Think dark green leafy veggies such as kale, Swiss chard, turnip greens, mustard greens, and collard greens (which all, ironically, have very strong spines), spinach, lettuce, watercress, bok choy, and brussels sprouts, as well as asparagus, okra, and peas.

• **Prebiotic fiber:** As you eat these foods, picture the calcium that you need to be strong, healthy, and sexy getting sucked up into your bones. That's what prebiotic fiber does. Asparagus, onions, chard, kale, artichokes, chicory, garlic, and leeks are all kings.

• **Vitamin D** promotes calcium absorption. You can consume all the calcium in the world, but without vitamin D it won't matter because you won't be able to absorb it. Calcium in your body without vitamin D is like being in a shopping mall without money; there are tons of things to buy, but you still leave empty-handed! Go for mushrooms. Maitake mushrooms lead the pack with a whopping 943 IU in an 84-gram serving ($1\frac{1}{4}$ cups), while one grilled portobello mushroom exposed to ultraviolet light has 493 IU. All mushrooms contain vitamin D, but growers can increase D levels by exposing the mushrooms to ultraviolet light. Like humans, mushrooms produce vitamin D after exposure to sunlight or a sunlamp. With mushrooms, their plant sterol, ergosterol, converts to vitamin D when exposed to light. With as little as five minutes of exposure to UV light, mushrooms can produce a substantial amount of vitamin D. Light-exposed mushrooms can provide close to 400 IU of vitamin D per serving (approximately four to five white button or crimini mushrooms, or one portobello).

Mushrooms stand out as the only source of vitamin D in the produce aisle and one of the few non-fortified food sources.

• **Potassium:** Potassium is like a parent who does whatever it takes to get food on the table. Potassium does what it takes to maintain homeostasis in the body, and in doing so helps to keep bone intact. Go for tomato products, potatoes, spinach, and sweet potatoes.

• **Magnesium:** Imagine being lost at sea and having a guide save you, leading you back to land. Magnesium plays this role for calcium, directing it to the bones. Your best magnesium bets? Spinach, beet greens, okra, tomato products, artichokes, plantains, potatoes, sweet potatoes, and collard greens and raisins (go for Curried Sweet Potato and Apple Salad, page 132, or Colorful Crunch Salad with Honey Dijon Vinaigrette, page 169). Beans, especially pinto, black, white, and kidney beans, are also a great way to get a boost of magnesium and even some calcium. Try our Hot Diggity Chili! (page 195) to warm up on a day when you're chilled to the bone.

• **Eat some olives.** New research reveals that hydroxytyrosol, an olive phytonutrient known for its role in helping to prevent cancer, can also help us prevent bone loss. A number of recent studies have found that consuming hydroxytyrosol and oleuropein, another key phytonutrient found in olives, increased calcium deposits in bone and decreased loss of total bone mass. Interestingly, the Mediterranean diet, which is rich in olives, is linked with a reduced risk of

osteoporosis—so perhaps olives are a major reason why!

> **Research has shown that walnuts —rich in alpha linolenic acid, an omega-3 fatty acid—decrease the rate of bone breakdown and keep bone formation constant. Other foods with alpha linolenic acid include flaxseed oil, ground flaxseeds, walnut oil, soybeans, soybean oil, and canola oil. Try our Muuuhr Muhammara Please (page 145) to get your dose.**

Spotlight on Peas

Recipes with Peas: Green Pea Hummus, page 137; Herbed Pea Soup with Spinach, page 165; Quinoa with Mixed Vegetables, page 193; Split Pea and Barley Soup, page 166

Pass the peas, please! When we started college we found ourselves making many of our meals and snacks at the dining hall's salad bar. It wasn't long before we created one of our favorite (and unusual) sweet snacks that tasted like a treat. We'd simply mix green peas and raisins. It wasn't until years afterward that we learned what a bone-alicious snack we had created. Peas and raisins for bones? You bet!

Most palates appreciate the sweet taste of peas before they even know that peas provide a triply sweet bone deal. First, on a basic bone-building front, green peas contain about 45 milligrams of calcium

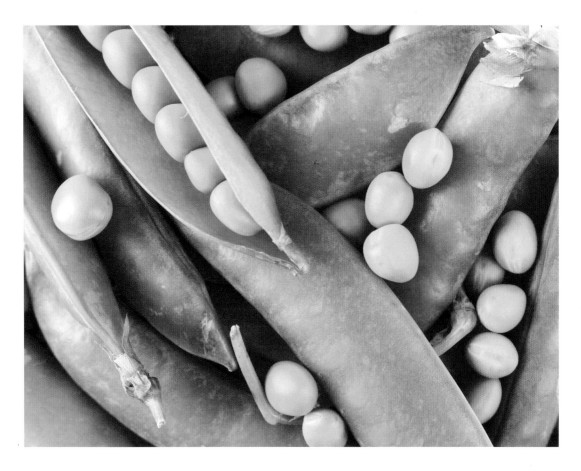

per cup to help keep those bones strong and sexy. Then, green peas are packed with nutrients that guard calcium—not just the calcium you consume from peas, but from all foods—ensuring that nothing can get in the way of calcium doing its job to keep your structure strong. The magnesium in peas helps calcium to find its way to your bones so calcium can do its work. The vitamin K helps to "glue" calcium to the bone, and peas' potassium protects the body from calcium loss. This combination is pretty incredible, given that most calcium-rich foods have nothing in them to help calcium to achieve its bone-building potential.

Making peas worthy of a second, third, fourth, and fifth bone-building helping is that they're a good source of bone-healthy copper, which plays a key role in the production of collagen, a component of bones and connective tissue. Peas' zinc supports healthy bone mass, and bone-healthy manganese is also no stranger to peas.

Another characteristic unique to peas? They're a good source of protein (most veggies are not). Protein helps build muscle mass, and strong bones and muscles keep each other stronger and healthier—and sexier!

If getting a strong, sexy structure isn't an enticing enough reason to eat your peas, consider that not only are peas bona fide bone strengtheners, they'll get you sexy in other ways too! Peas have impressive amounts of fiber and protein (per cup, about 8 to 10 grams of each) that directly control the speed at which we digest our food, causing a gradual pace of digestion and breakdown of starches into sugars, ultimately helping blood sugar levels to be steady. This will keep energy levels high and stable and will prevent mood swings. Now, that's ap*pea*ling. What's more, peas have a low glycemic index, and in combination with their unique anti-inflammatory properties, phytonutrient content, and high fiber and protein content, they help to provide excellent blood sugar control and protect against diabetes.

Add that peas are an excellent source of vitamin C to keep your immune system strong and vitamin A for beautiful skin and vision. They are also a good source of heart-healthy fiber and folate, and they are associated with a decreased risk of stomach cancer, so we expect you'll be keeping our Green Pea Hummus on hand so you can dip your baby carrots, celery sticks, or toasted pita into it every day.

Did you know that peas are actually members of the legume family? And they're one of the few legumes that are commonly sold as fresh vegetables, unlike other members of the legume family like lentils, chickpeas, and beans that are usually sold in the dried form.

Spotlight on Turnip Greens

Recipes with Turnip Greens (simply substitute turnip greens for cooked spinach in any of the following recipes): Creamy Spinach Dip, page 134; Easy Spinach Pomodoro, page 214; Herbed Pea Soup with Spinach, page 165; Simple Sautéed Spinach, page 234; Spinach Squares, page 154; Tomato, Spinach, Egg 'n' Feta Never Tasted Betta Wrap, page 123

We didn't grow up eating turnip greens, and in fact, when we first bought turnips, we cut off the greens and chucked them out, keeping only the turnip bulb, believing that was the prize. And then we moved to the South. Southerners love their greens, from collards to mustard greens to kale, and that's where we first tried turnip greens. We're thankful we did, and we're never turning back. After trying our Simple Sautéed Turnip Greens (aka Spinach) recipe, y'all won't, either. Although southerners traditionally season their turnip greens with salt pork, this isn't how we eat 'em. We're huge fans of using just a little bit of olive oil, garlic, a dash of salt and pepper, and hot pepper sauce. When eaten raw, the leaves are pungent and slightly bitter, but cook them and they become milder, and you can substitute them for cooked spinach in any of our recipes. Substitute turnip greens for the spinach in our Herbed Pea Soup with Spinach, which is to die for. Your taste buds will thank you, and so will your bones, with this double bone boost from the peas and turnip greens both.

Ironically, turnip greens have a really strong spine, just like the sexy one they help you to attain. Just one cup of cooked turnip greens has a whopping 200 milligrams of calcium—and you get all of that calcium in just 30 calories. Even if you were drinking nonfat milk, you'd have to have to swallow double the calories for the same amount of calcium.

Wanna make sure all that calcium actually gets cemented to your bones? Thanks to turnip greens' excellent vitamin K content, they'll take care of that for you—with an extraordinary 661 percent of your daily need in one cup! And turnip greens don't stop there. These greens are also an excellent source of vitamin C and copper, which both play a key role in the production of collagen, that essential component of bones and connective tissue. Not to mention,

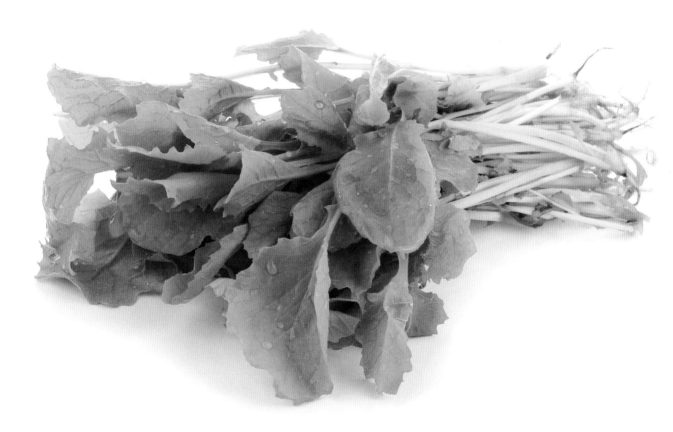

turnip greens are a terrific source of manganese, which is needed to form bone. In fact, turnip greens put all their bone-building cards on the table (or shall we say plate?), offering a very good source of potassium to prevent calcium loss from the body as well as containing lots of magnesium to help usher all of that calcium to your bones!

More Reasons You Shouldn't Turnip the Chance to Eat Turnip Greens

We've all heard that we need to eat more veggies in the cruciferous family like broccoli, kale, cauliflower, and brussels sprouts, since they're packed with nutrients. Did you know that turnip greens also are part of the family? Cruciferous veggies are known for being potent cancer fighters. One reason why they are so potent is that their glucosinolate content can be converted into the potential cancer-preventative phytonutrient isothiocyanates (ITCs). Turns out turnip greens are higher in glucosinolates than cabbage, kale, cauliflower, and broccoli. In turnip greens the strongest links are to the prevention of cancers of the bladder, breasts, colon, lungs, prostate, and ovaries. Turnip greens have a strong role in the body's detox system, its antioxidant system, and its inflammatory/anti-inflammatory system—and these are all also important in the prevention of cancer.

What's more, turnip greens help to keep your heart and digestive system healthy and are an excellent source of vitamin A (in the form of beta-carotene), vitamin E, vitamin B_6, folate, and fiber. Turnip greens are a very good source of iron and vitamin B_2 and a good source of phosphorus, vitamin B_1, vitamin B_3, vitamin B_5, omega-3 fatty acids, and protein.

Although turnip greens do contain oxalates, which bind to calcium and can prevent its absorption, research shows that the level of oxalates is low in turnip greens and that you can still reap the benefits, including calcium absorption.

To Get the Most Nutrition and Flavor per Turnip Green Bite

After washing turnip greens under cold running water, cut them into half-inch slices to help them to cook quickly and evenly. Then let them sit for at least five minutes before cooking. Sprinkle with lemon juice before letting them sit, to help activate their myrosinase enzymes and increase formation of beneficial cancer-fighting isothiocyanates. Then steam them for five minutes.

CHAPTER 6

The Slim & Trim Factor

Veggies to Lose Weight Fast

The Problem: You need to lose weight quickly. You know better than to try a crash diet, because you don't want the weight loss to be fleeting, but you don't know how to lose weight quickly without the pounds piling back on.

Here's What You Need: More vegetables! Especially non-starchy fiber-packed vegetables—raw, cooked, or in soups—that you can fill up on at meals, for snacks, and before dinner parties and cocktail events. These veggies will limit your intake of high-calorie foods and prevent you from overeating or filling up on other unhealthy items. Some of the best weight-loss veggies are cabbage, cucumbers, cauliflower, bok choy, fennel, celery, bell peppers, broccoli, mushrooms, turnips, string beans, carrots, and leafy greens like spinach, kale, and turnip greens. Indulge in our Roasted Turnip Nips (page 151) and you'll never need a high-calorie snack food again.

Here's Why: Veggies are a dieter's dream come true, especially non-starchy fiber-packed vegetables, which are low in calories and high in vitamins, minerals, phytonutrients, water, and fiber. Fill your plate with them and you have less room for the foods that expand your waist and hips. Fiber-packed vegetables fill your stomach with fiber, not calories. Plus, they fill your stomach with water and nutrients. So they make you full, not fat. If you get enough fiber, research shows, you actually will absorb as much as 90 fewer calories a day. This equals a 10-pound weight loss this year alone! And that's the weight you can lose before you even start replacing high-calorie foods with vegetables. That bikini is already fitting better.

Want to take the edge off hunger? Fill up on veggies or veggie soup. These are your pre-meal secret weapons, so you don't overeat at social dinners, cocktail parties, or meals. They are very low in calories, and research shows that when you eat soup as a first course, you eat roughly 20 percent fewer calories at your meal.

Spotlight on Cabbage (Green, Red, Savoy) and Bok Choy

Recipes with Cabbage and Bok Choy: Asian Lettuce Wrap with Hoisin-Ginger Dipping Sauce, page 170;

Bengali Cabbage, page 205; Dieter's Delight Chock Full of Veggies Soup, page 163; Just Call Me Baby Bok Choy, page 228; Ole! Mexican Cabbage with Black Beans and Avocados, page 179; Red Cabbage Salad with Grapes and Ginger Dressing, page 180

In addition to red, green, and savoy cabbage, there is bok choy, also known as Chinese cabbage. Related to kale, broccoli, collards, and brussels sprouts, cabbage is a member of the cruciferous vegetable family. When it comes to weight loss, all varieties of cabbage are stellar, and we'll be using them interchangeably as we refer to their weight loss attributes.

As we are identical twins, our entire life people have wanted to know how they can tell us apart. When we were four years old, people would ask us this question and Lyssie would say, "I'm the one who likes cabbage." Tammy actually liked cabbage too, but was shyer and typically afraid to speak up for herself. The truth is, even at four, cabbage was part of our lives, and it still is today. We're not sure if it's because we're part Hungarian, but we both love purple cabbage and eat it daily. And when the Cabbage Soup Diet that promised "10 pounds lost in seven days" became the craze, we thought that the soup sounded delicious despite realizing that it was part of a crash diet that would have fleeting results.

How ironic that cabbage is round and heavy when it can make you lean and light. And you don't have to exist solely on cabbage soup to reap its weight-loss benefits. Here's why: Cabbage is one of the lowest-calorie foods. One entire cup of raw cabbage adds just 17 fat-and-cholesterol-free calories to your daily total, and just 33 calories per cup when cooked (cooked is more compact than raw)—less than the amount of calories in a single teaspoon of oil. However, its incredibly low calorie count is just a piece of what makes cabbage the total slenderizing package.

Combine that minuscule amount of calories in a cup-size serving with 3 grams of fiber and lots of water. In fact, 92 percent of cabbage is water. This means that cabbage fills you up with water and fiber and virtually no calories. Imagine being hungry. Think of some of the fiber in cabbage as a sponge that expands in your stomach when water is added, so it takes up a lot of space, filling your stomach so you feel less hungry and eat less, helping to shrink your waist. Cabbage does this while keeping you hydrated. Plus, it's loaded with nutrients that keep you strong and healthy so that your body can perform properly—this includes adequately digesting your food and keeping your metabolism speedy and running at full throttle. Cabbage is a dieter's dream come true!

Pushing cabbage over the edge as a weight-loss star is its versatility—it can easily be incorporated in main and side dishes. This means that it attacks a thick waistline in two ways. First, it fills you up with very few calories (while providing bountiful nutrients!) so you eat less. Then it replaces higher-calorie fare by

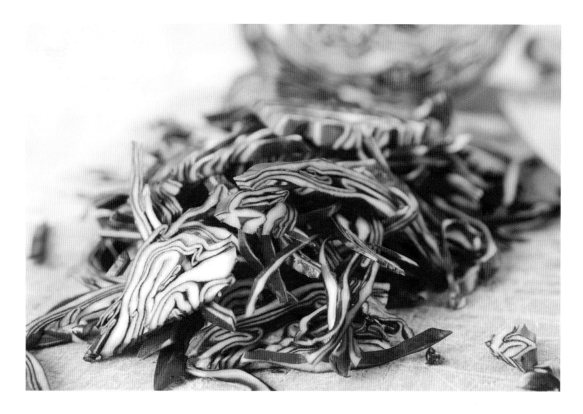

taking the place of practically any food in most dishes. Think of it this way: The same one-cup portion of spaghetti and meatballs has about 275 calories. That's more than eight times as many calories as that same portion of cooked cabbage! Replace just one cup of spaghetti and meatballs on your plate (most people eat two to three cups at a sitting) by mixing in cabbage. Do this daily and you'll get a delicious flavor and wonderful texture, and you'll lose two pounds this month. Ditto for chinese beef and fried rice (except you'll lose four pounds!). Same goes for chicken pot pie. And you're still eating the food you love plus getting the yummy cabbage. Want to lose weight?

Look no further than our Bengali Cabbage—a half-cup serving has fewer than 50 calories.

Other Health Bonuses in the Cabbage Patch

One of the reasons that cabbage is the perfect weight-loss food is because it is nutrient rich. Cabbage is an excellent source of bone-healthy vitamin K, manganese, and calcium and heart-healthy folate and potassium. Although cabbage is not a fatty food, it provides the omega-3 fatty acid alpha-linolenic acid (ALA). This may be one of the reasons cabbage offers powerful anti-inflammatory benefits. Cabbage is an antioxidant powerhouse, as its vitamin C helps to keep your immune system strong and healthy and protect your cells against damage. Additionally, cabbage is packed with phytonutrients that make it a mighty force when it comes to detoxification, keeping the digestive tract lining healthy and fighting cancer, heart disease, and diseases related to inflammation.

Spotlight on Celery

Recipes with Celery: Dieter's Delight Chock Full of Veggies Soup, page 163; Edamame and Corn Salad, page 173; Fennel Stuffed Potatoes, page 189; Green-ana Apple Pear Smoothie, page 109; Split Pea and Barley Soup, page 166; Stuffed Celery Bites, page 155; Vegetable Broth, page 164

Our earliest celery memories date back to when we were little kids. We would play in the sandbox and then come inside for a snack of what our Mom called "frogs on a log." There were two kinds—the logs stuffed with peanut butter and raisins (frogs), and the ones stuffed with cream cheese and raisins. Regardless, the logs were always the same, crunchy celery sticks with their tunnels filled, and they were so much fun to eat. Have your kids try for themselves! (See our Ribb—it! Frogs on a Celery-Rib Log, page 150).

Ironically, although the log's filling wasn't exactly low calorie, the celery log itself is one of the best weight-loss foods.

Long, slim, and firm, just like it can help you to be, celery's so low in calories you may have even heard that it has negative calories. Although that's not entirely true, the calories are extremely low—a single four-inch stalk of celery contains just 1 calorie! It takes more calories to digest it than it contains, and that's partially thanks to all of its fiber. Celery contains 2 grams of fiber in a mere 17 calories' worth, and in just 100 calories of celery you get 11.5 grams of fiber—almost half of what you need in an entire day. Consider that fiber fills you up and, since you can't digest it, actually pulls some calories out with it when it leaves your body. When you fill up on this very low-calorie food, think of all those calories you're not consuming! Nice work, Slim!

What's more, celery is 95 percent water. This is critical for your weight loss. Water fills your stomach without any calories, so you feel less hungry and you eat less. And it's needed to keep you hydrated, so that your body can perform properly—this includes the proper metabolism and digestion of your food. When you lose weight, you need water to flush out all of the end products of fat metabolism, including the toxins stored in the fat cells. Celery helps you to lose fat and aids in flushing it out.

Hungry? Our clients always ask what they can eat when they just want to crunch on something mindlessly. Celery is the answer. If you're someone who eats because you're stressed, celery is for you.

Celery offers a great crunch, and because it's so low in calories, you can eat as much as you want. Keep washed and trimmed celery stalks in a plastic bag in the fridge, and as hunger or cravings strike during the day, simply eat a couple of stalks to quash your appetite. Dip celery in low-calorie salsa or in dips (say hello to our Artichoke Hummus, page 126, and our Creamy Spinach Dip, page 134) so you don't get tired of eating the celery on its own. Go for our Stuffed Celery Bites or our Dieter's Delight soup.

And because celery is so low in calories, it's a great food to add to other foods and to combine in meals to add flavor and bulk to the meal with fewer calories. You can do this with soups, stews, casseroles, and healthy stir-fries. You'll eat less high-calorie fare and more celery, drastically cutting the calories you consume and your pants size. Thank you, celery! It not only thins out the calories, but your waist too!

The secret to celery's weight-loss success is simply to eat a lot of it. In the process, you'll fill up on it, swallow very few calories while consuming all of its health-promoting nutrients, and displace the higher-calorie foods from your diet. Watch the pounds melt away.

There's More to Celery than Slimming

What's more, as you celery-size your waist and hips, you'll boost your health. Celery is an excellent source of vitamin K; without vitamin K you'll have weak bones and your blood won't be able to clot or form a scab. Celery also is packed with antioxidants that protect your body against disease and keep your skin healthy. It's a very good source of dietary fiber, to keep your digestive tract in good shape and fight against disease. Its potassium will help to keep your blood pressure healthy, while its B vitamins (B_1, B_2, B_5, B_6) will help to keep your energy revved. The calcium and magnesium in celery make it good for bone health. The phytonutrients in celery help in the prevention of cancer, and in combating high blood pressure, high cholesterol, heart disease, and stroke.

CHAPTER 7

The Perk-Up Factor

Veggies for Energy

The Problem: You're tired, so you rely on caffeine from your morning coffee or from an afternoon soda to give you a boost. You often crash after lunch and crave a candy bar or something else sugary or with caffeine for a pick-me-up. After giving in to your craving, you get an energy high followed by a crash. You want to feel energetic naturally without relying on stimulants.

Here's What You Need: Quality, high-fiber carbohydrates like whole grains, fruits, and vegetables, particularly one-quarter to one-half cup of a higher-carbohydrate veggie like peas, potatoes, corn, butternut squash, or other winter squash combined with protein at mealtimes. We'll focus on the veggies here.

Here's Why: Starchy vegetables . . .

• **provide nutrient-rich complex carbohydrates** that fuel your brain, your muscles, and your central nervous system. They are your body's energy source.

• **are loaded with B vitamins and magnesium** to help turn your food

into usable energy so that you feel invigorated and refreshed.

• **are a good source of water,** which is necessary for energy. Plus, every process in the body relies on water. Without adequate water from food, dehydration is likely and you will feel exhausted.

• **are packed with antioxidants** that help to rid your body of damaging toxins that break the body down, tax the system, and wear you out.

• **often contain copper,** which is needed to produce energy.

• **contain potassium** to keep your blood pressure in check and your heart in better working condition so that it can easily pump nutrient-rich, oxygen-carrying blood throughout your body to energize you.

Spotlight on Butternut Squash

Recipes with Butternut Squash: Butternut and Turnip Barley Risotto, page 185; Butternut Squash and Mango Mash, page 210. Recipes with Pumpkin: Pumpkin Cream Cheese Muffins, page 149;

The Perk-Up Factor

Pumpkin 'n' Apple-y Yogurt Parfait, page 118; Pumpkin Pancakes, page 117; Sweet and Savory Pumpkin Quiche, page 120. Note: Butternut Squash and Pumpkin are very similar in nutritional benefits.

We were about four years old when we had our first encounter with butternut squash. We were at the grocery store with our mom, hanging on to her for dear life as we always did, being painfully shy kids. We spotted the butternut squash and begged Mom to buy the "biggest pear we'd ever seen." Mom, who had never made butternut squash, convinced us to settle for "real" pears instead. Years later we tried butternut squash for the first time in college, and we were disappointed to have missed out on this sweet flavor for so many years.

We also missed out on one of the best energy-boosting veggies out there, and we certainly could have utilized butternut squash when we had a long school day followed by a soccer game and speed-skating practice, to keep our energy level kicked into high gear.

Without carbohydrates, exhaustion sets in. Your brain can't focus. You lack concentration. Your memory suffers. Your muscles feel weak and fatigued. Your coordination seems off. Every little movement becomes difficult. Making matters worse, many people are trying to limit carbohydrates like breads, so they really feel drained and crave a pick-me-up. Good news! If you eat butternut squash, this doesn't happen. Your body receives its much needed carbohydrates

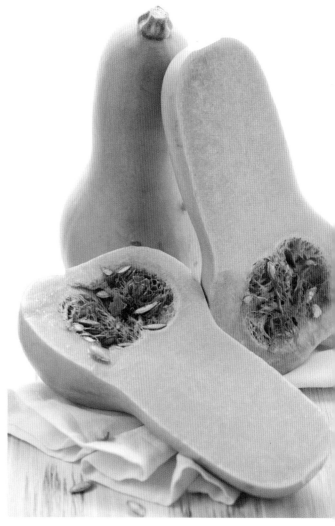

and you get an energy boost. Unlike the carbs in white bread or other refined carbohydrates, those in squash arrive in your body packaged with fiber, which slows the rate at which they enter the bloodstream. You get a continual release of energy, keeping your mood stable and extending the energy boost without crashes. Each cup of baked winter squash provides 22 percent of your daily fiber need, ensuring a long-lasting rejuvenation so that

45

you may never need that cup of coffee again. If you need to concentrate for a big presentation, a test, or a meeting, butternut squash is the veggie for you. Preparing to compete in a race or hit the gym? Go for butternut squash.

Most people don't realize that a dip in hydration of even 1 to 2 percent makes you sluggish. In hydration, 1 to 2 percent is a big deal; by the time you are slightly thirsty, your energy level is already affected. People don't realize that they feel tired because they are dehydrated. It's not just what you drink that contributes to your hydration, but also what you eat—at least 20 percent, and much more if you eat your fruits and veggies. Like most vegetables, butternut squash is high in water, about 86 percent, so eating it can help to protect against the sluggishness that results from dehydration. Your cells rely on water for every process in the body, so eat your butternut squash and you'll prevent dehydration and the associated exhaustion—and as an added bonus you'll prevent your skin from looking dry and weathered.

More energy-boosting props to butternut squash! It's loaded with magnesium, which turns the food that you eat into energy. Think of generating energy like driving a car. If you don't have the key to turn on the engine, you won't be able to start the car and you won't be able to drive. Similarly, if you don't have magnesium, you won't be able to start the chain reactions that generate energy, and you will feel exhausted, weak, and unable

to move. You'll also be prone to muscle cramps and charley horses. If you've ever experienced either, you know how exhausting they can be. Our clients who wake up with muscle cramps find that if they boost their magnesium intake, they make these muscle spasms a problem of their past, along with the exhaustion and crankiness that accompany them.

Good-bye, cup o' joe! You've been traded in for a cup of our Butternut and Turnip Barley Risotto. Who needs caffeine when squash has got vitamin B_6, vitamin B_2 (riboflavin), and folate? Vitamin B_6 and riboflavin are essential to get energy from the food you eat. Riboflavin is particularly important for energy for the heart and skeletal muscles. Without enough folate, the production of red blood cells decreases. When your red blood cell count is low, the distribution of oxygen throughout the body is disrupted. This is when fatigue and weakness can set in. Not gonna happen to you—butternut squash will help you stay strong and invigorated.

Although you may think that's the last of butternut squash's perks, it's also got copper. This material used to make pennies is also needed to produce energy. Copper helps the body absorb iron, and it works with iron to form red blood cells. Without enough red blood cells, exhaustion sets in. To prevent this, look no further than butternut squash.

Antioxidants are scavengers for those toxins and chemicals that tax our bodies, leave us feeling fatigued, and lead to disease. Vitamin C is a potent antioxidant, and butternut squash is an excellent source of it. One cup of baked butternut squash contains nearly 33 percent of your daily need for vitamin C. So vitamin C nips fatigue in the bud; if the toxins aren't able to create damage, it's not an option for exhaustion to be a side effect. Hello, Butternut Squash and Mango Mash, good-bye, afternoon slump.

Other Benefits of Eating Butternut Squash

Butternut squash also is an excellent source of immune-supportive vitamin A. The fiber in the butternut squash promotes digestive health and regularity, and its pectin makes it a powerful anti-inflammatory. Folate, omega-3 fatty acids, B vitamins, magnesium, and potassium make butternut squash very heart healthy. Lastly, the copper and vitamin K make butternut squash a good bone builder.

> **Trying to get into better shape? Get more butternut squash by subbing it for the sweet potato in our Coco Sweet Potatoes with Mango Salsa (page 130) or in our Curried Sweet Potato and Apple Salad (page 132). A study out from the U.S. Department of Agriculture found that women who fell short of their daily quota for magnesium tired more quickly during a jog than those who consumed sufficient amounts.**

Spotlight on Potatoes

Recipes with Potatoes: Fennel Stuffed Potatoes, page 189; Garlic and Herb Potato Stacks, page 136; Potato Bites, page 230; Sriracha Potato Cha Cha, page 236

Growing up, we loved to run through our neighborhood, racing each other, playing tag or Capture the Flag, or dashing through the creek in our backyard for a little adventure. We'd go nonstop until Mom rang the dinner bell that hung on our back porch to signify it was mealtime. As we grew older and went to high school, we focused our energy on soccer, cross-country running, and speed skating. The night before our big soccer games, our team would get together for "carb parties," where we'd eat foods that supposedly gave us energy and made us perform better. Typically the team would enjoy pasta dinners, and occasionally potatoes. The night before our team made the county finals, we had fueled up on potatoes. Never had we played so well as a team, or as individuals. From that day on, we all credited the potatoes, and they became our "energy-boosting meal choice." After learning about how potatoes rev energy, it's no wonder they worked their magic.

If you need energy, potatoes are the perfect fuel to rev your engine. Potatoes are one of the best, most nutritious sources of carbohydrates. The carbohydrates in potatoes fuel your brain, your muscles, and your nervous system.

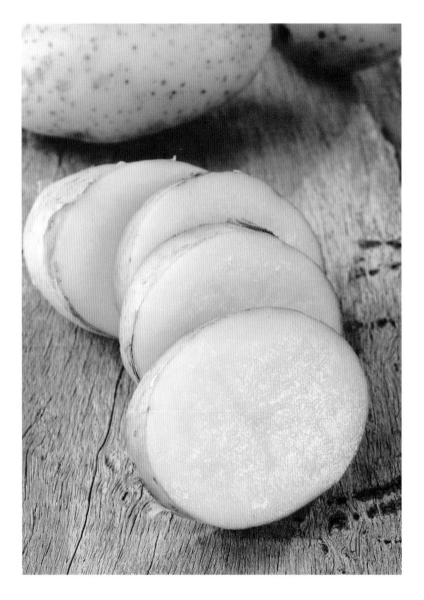

Without these carbohydrates, you'd feel miserable and lifeless. Consume a potato at lunchtime and, thanks to the carbohydrates and the nearly 3 grams of fiber in just a small potato, you'll sail through your day. That's because the fiber won't allow you to crash; it will extend the energy boost of the carbohydrates and keep it stable.

Potatoes are a rich source of vitamin B_6. One cup of baked potato contains 21 percent of the daily value for this important nutrient. Vitamin B_6 is necessary for the breakdown of glycogen, the form in which sugar is stored in our muscle cells and liver, so it's critical when it comes to athletic performance and endurance, when you need to tap into an energy supply to fuel you. Since vitamin B_6 turns the food that you eat into energy, it's a key player when it comes to fighting fatigue and having brain and muscle energy to power through your day. Without B_6, you'd feel weak and exhausted. The same goes for magnesium, copper, and the B vitamins riboflavin, niacin, folate, and thiamin, all of which the body needs to create energy. This hot potato doesn't short-circuit here either. Need an energy surge? Bite no further than our Garlic and Herb Potato Stacks.

The energy boost created by a potato doesn't end there. Potatoes are one of the best sources of potassium in the produce section. For fluids to fully penetrate and hydrate cells, you need potassium. The mineral is also important for muscle and nerve function, which is key to energize the muscles. Potassium also keeps you energized by keeping your blood pressure down so that your heart can function at its peak and swiftly deliver oxygen-rich blood throughout your body and to your extremities. Without enough potassium, your heart will have to work in overdrive, and it will leave you feeling as if the wind was knocked out of you. You'll want to take a nap, and you won't want to get up.

Potatoes are an excellent source of vitamin C, with a cup of baked potato providing 27.7 percent of the vitamin C you need in a day. Vitamin C destroys toxins that damage our bodies, break us down, and leave us worn out. Think of vitamin C coming to save the day and giving you that second wind; it's your secret weapon that picks you up and springs you into a high-powered running mode, just when you thought you'd have to hit the hay midday. Sriracha Potato Cha Cha, anyone?

This Spud's for You

Potatoes are superstars when it comes to an energy boost, but their benefits don't end there. Potatoes are an antioxidant powerhouse, rivaling the nutrients in broccoli. They contain a variety of phytonutrients including carotenoids, flavonoids (especially potent when it comes to fighting heart disease, cancer, and other chronic diseases), and caffeic acid. Potatoes also contain patatin, which helps keep harmful free radicals from wreaking havoc in our bodies and creating destruction, aging, and disease. Potatoes' vitamin C, folic acid, quercitin, and kukoamines are key players in lowering blood pressure; kukoamines have been found in only one other plant, the goji berry.

Storage Tip: Don't store your spuds in the refrigerator. Their starch will turn to sugar, and they won't taste good. Store them in a burlap bag away from onions. Both onions and potatoes will emit gases that will cause them both to degrade.

CHAPTER 8

Skin Dulgence

Veggies That Are Better than Anti-Wrinkle Cream

The Problem: Your skin is lackluster, broken out, or shows unwanted signs of aging.

What You Need: Omega-3 fatty acids and a large variety of antioxidants like vitamin C, beta-carotene, vitamin E, and others, a.k.a. the skin fillers, plumpers, and Botox of the food kingdom.

Here's Why: Vitamin C keeps skin youthful and elastic by aiding in collagen formation. Beta-carotene helps give a healthy glow and hue while protecting skin from sun damage. Antioxidants guard against premature aging by helping to prevent cell damage, including that from pollution and other environmental toxins, stress, and the sun. Omega-3s contain powerful anti-inflammatory compounds that give skin a smoother appearance. Water-rich vegetables and those packed with potassium keep the skin hydrated so it doesn't look wrinkled and withered.

Here's How to Get It: Vitamin C is in tomatoes, cucumbers, bell peppers, broccoli, and potatoes; find beta-carotene in carrots, spinach, sweet potatoes, butternut squash, and other orange- and green-colored produce; Omega-3s are in cabbage; antioxidants and anti-inflammation compounds are found in all veggies, particularly the ones we spotlight.

Spotlight on Tomatoes

Recipes with Tomatoes (which are so versatile that we have 25 recipes with them; here are a few where they costar): Eggplant Parmesan, page 187; Golden Gazpacho in Petite Cucumber Cradles, page 139; Guacamole Stuffed Tomato Poppers, page 140; Italian Mushrooms, Tomato, and Spinach, page 224; Mediterranean Pizza, page 192; Roasted Tomato Puttanesca, page 199; Rockin' Ratatouille, page 152; Spaghetti Squash with Fresh Tomato Sauce, page 200; Tomato Artichoke Pasta Bake, page 201; Tomato and Basil Bruschetta, page 157; Tomato, Spinach, Egg 'n' Feta Never Tasted Betta Wrap, page 123

You'd probably assume that when we, two registered dietitians, think of tomatoes, it's their powerful nutrients that come to mind first. Not so. For us, summertime immediately pops to mind, and we reminisce about growing up and devouring luscious, juicy, vibrantly red beefsteak tomatoes drizzled with olive oil and sweet balsamic as if they were candy, or devouring our mom's hearty homemade tomato sauce. As much as we are focused on the flavor of the delicious tomato, it actually comes second to the health attributes and the benefits that tomatoes provide for the skin.

Tomatoes are a powerhouse of antioxidants like vitamin C, beta-carotene, and lycopene. In just one cup of raw tomato you get 38 percent of the Daily Value (DV)—your daily need—of vitamin C and 29.9 percent of the DV for vitamin A. Although most of us think of vitamin C as the flu-fighting vitamin, it does much more than this, especially when it comes to our skin. Vitamin C is needed for growth and repair for all tissues in our body, including the skin. If you have any type of skin wound or flaw, think of vitamin C as your ambulance and medical crew. Imagine vitamin C rushing to the wound with stupendous powers to hasten healing. Then imagine vitamin C protecting that wound, acting as your medicated Band-Aid, shielding your skin against foreign invaders like free radicals, which age and damage your skin. Load up on tomatoes to fight age spots, wrinkles, and blemishes.

When it comes to your skin, perhaps vitamin C's most important job is aiding in the production of collagen. Collagen keeps skin firm and tight and improves the appearance of wrinkles by keeping skin elastic. Tomatoes are your Botox, but without the needles.

Beta-carotene and lycopene both are potent antioxidants that protect

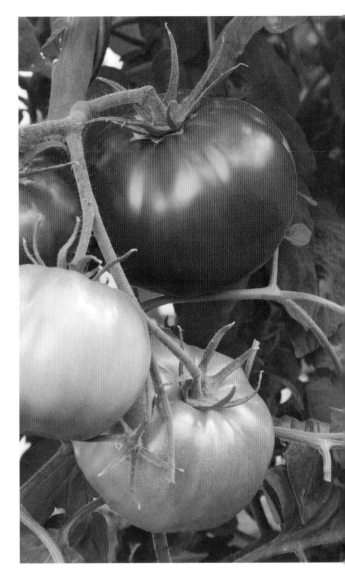

skin against the sun's harmful rays. It's the damaging rays of the sun that are responsible for premature wrinkles, freckles, sunspots, and cancer. Tomatoes serve as your sunscreen without the messy lotion (although we do recommend a sunscreen with an SPF of 15 or higher as well).

Acne sufferers too can rejoice, as tomatoes' beta-carotene is a gold mine for them—also offering anti-inflammatory benefits by reducing the swelling of their inflamed skin. If it were possible to swallow your sunscreen and your acne medication together, our Spaghetti Squash with Fresh Tomato Sauce, Guacamole Stuffed Tomato Poppers, and Tomato Artichoke Pasta Bake are your ticket.

The beta-carotene in tomatoes is converted into vitamin A in the body, and it aids in the development of skin cells. Rejuvenating old skin and building new skin is what will keep your skin young and looking refreshed. Vitamin A also helps to strengthen skin; when skin is strong, it won't wrinkle as easily or show age. Weak, thin skin shows wrinkles and age.

Tomatoes are 94 percent water, so they are a true skin hydrator. Dehydrated skin looks sunken, wrinkled, damaged, and old. Tomatoes prevent this. The water in tomatoes fills the spaces between skin cells and plumps the skin up. Plus, they are a very good source of potassium, which also helps to hydrate your skin. Tomatoes are your injectable fillers—but, again, without the needles.

No Such Thing as a Rotten Tomato

Sure, tomatoes appear to have magical powers when it comes to skin, but their benefits don't end there. Intake of tomatoes is linked to everything from fighting heart disease to slowing the aging process. The lycopene in tomatoes fights numerous kinds of cancer, including prostate cancer, and also appears to be important in bone health. Diets that include tomatoes have been linked to a reduced risk of obesity as well as of Alzheimer's disease and other neurological disorders.

Spotlight on Cucumbers

Recipes with Cucumbers: Cold Cucumber and Avocado Soup, page 160; Colorful Crunch Salad with Honey Dijon Vinaigrette, page 169; Fruity Green Smoothie, page 108; Golden Gazpacho in Petite Cucumber Cradles, page 139; Minted Mango Melon Detox Smoothie, page 111; Mojito Salad, page 178; Sparkling Cucumber Detox and Refresher, page 113

It was during the summer after our freshman year of high school that we truly started to enjoy cucumbers. We'd train for soccer, practicing in the hot sun before riding our bikes to the pool to cool off. We'd eat our brown-bagged lunch under a tree in the shade. We had discovered the refreshing cool crunch of the cucumber in a whole grain pita pocket, and we'd pack our sandwiches (tuna, turkey, cheese, hummus) high with cucumber slices. There was something refreshing and revitalizing about those crunchy, cool, and delicious bites, and we really looked forward to eating them as we recovered from a tough workout.

Since then, it seems that every time we go for a rejuvenating massage or facial, there is a cucumber face mask or lotion or even cucumber-infused water at the spa, as cucumber has become the universal symbol of calm, rejuvenation, and healing. And when you understand what cucumber has to offer, it's no surprise that it's known for being so restorative, especially for your skin.

Cucumbers are 96 percent water. It's only natural they are so thirst-quenching! They provide almost as much fluid as pure water, yet they also saturate your cells with skin-enhancing nutrients. They start by filling the cells beneath your skin, plumping the skin up and making it look youthful. So as cucumbers hydrate, they smooth the skin while helping it to appear lush, dewy, and glowing. Combine this with cucumber's hydrating mineral, potassium, and you've got yourself some luxurious skin.

After diving into our Mojito Salad, which is chock-full of cucumbers and watermelon, your skin will really be at its best. Cucumbers (and watermelon!) contain skin-enhancing carotenoids. Carotenoids give faces a sun-kissed hue, but without the harmful rays of the sun. And faces with this hint of orange are

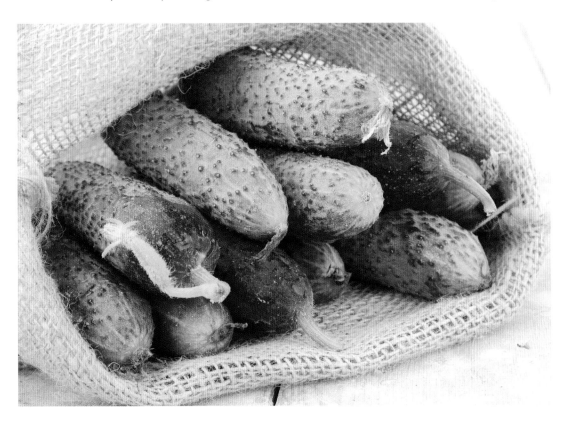

perceived as healthier and more attractive. Au revoir, lackluster skin!

Adding to cucumber's skin rejuvenation capability is vitamin C, a potent antioxidant that plays a big part in collagen synthesis. Collagen makes skin strong, elastic, and stretchy. Imagine having skin like a baby's that returns to its original position after making expressions. Vitamin C helps the skin to do this. Want smoother skin? Why pay for pricey dermatological procedures when cucumber is the answer?

Cucumbers also beautify your skin with both their antioxidant (vitamin C, beta-carotene, and manganese) and anti-inflammatory (vitamin K) phytonutrients and many other nontraditional nutrients like flavonoids that decelerate the aging process. Damage from everyday living (stress, environmental pollution, UV light rays, and more) occurs in the form of free radicals that lead to wrinkles, aged skin, and inflammation, which makes skin look stressed and full of blemishes. Bite into a cucumber to be on your way to prevent this.

Although cucumbers work endlessly as your skin's beauty potion from the inside out, their benefits go on. Cucumbers also boast heart-healthy potassium and magnesium, bone-fortifying manganese, and pantothenic acid (vitamin B_5) to help you get your energy from food. Thanks to all of their anti-inflammatory and antioxidant nutrients, cucumbers help to fight cancer. In fact, cucumbers contain numerous specific anticancer nutrients including cucurbitacins, which block several different pathways that cancer thrives on. And if protecting your skin and body isn't enough, cucumbers also contain the important nail-health-promoting mineral silica. Join us for some Cold Cucumber and Avocado Soup!

CHAPTER 9

A Bun (Loaded with Veggies) in the Oven

Veggies for a Healthy Pregnancy

The Problem: Even before many women are pregnant, they don't get enough of the important nutrients they need for their childbearing years, and when they're pregnant they have an even harder time meeting the increased nutrient needs for the growth and development of the baby.

Here's What You Need: Nutrients that nourish the "baby's home" for the next nine months—namely, YOU! You need nutrients that not only create a healthy environment for the baby to live in, but that also aid in the baby's growth and development. Consume plenty of veggies like asparagus, soybeans, sweet potatoes, spinach, and lettuce that help you meet your requirements for folic acid (folate) and other B vitamins, calcium, iron, vitamin A, fiber, and antioxidants like vitamin C and vitamin E.

Here's Why: Getting adequate folic acid aids in the growth of the placenta and prevents abnormalities of the baby's brain and spine, while other B vitamins are critical for the development of healthy skin, eyes, and nerves. Iron is needed for growth of the baby and placenta and to deliver oxygen to your baby.

Calcium helps your baby to have strong teeth and bones, a healthy heart, nerves, and muscles, and to develop a normal heartbeat and blood-clotting abilities. If you don't get enough, you draw on the calcium stores in your own bones, putting them at risk for osteoporosis. Vitamin A, too, is needed for the development of bones and teeth. Antioxidants like vitamin C and E protect you and your baby against free radical damage. Fiber helps keep moms comfortable by fighting constipation.

Spotlight on Asparagus

Recipes with Asparagus: Baby Bellas and Asparagus, page 206; Floating Asparagus Rafts, page 215; Heavenly Roasted Vegetables, page 219

When Tammy was pregnant with her twins, she was quite disappointed during her first trimester to find that the simple thought of many of her favorite pre-pregnancy veggies made her nauseous. Knowing how important the nutrients in vegetables are for a healthy pregnancy, she was hoping she would somehow be the lucky one who was immune to morning sickness. And although she felt very

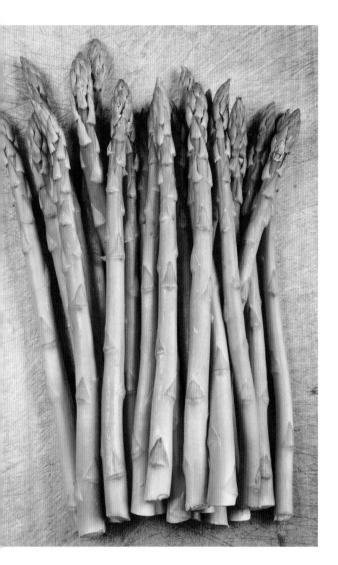

prepare it with an Asian flair. If there's any truth to the hypothesis that you crave what your body needs, this makes a good case for it!

Asparagus is the veggie to call for all things baby. The first thing your doctor will tell you about your pregnancy is to be sure to get enough folic acid to help support the growth of the placenta and to prevent spina bifida and other neural tube defects. At 88 micrograms per half-cup serving of boiled asparagus, asparagus is a real superstar when it comes to folic acid, ranking among the highest of the vegetables and helping you to meet your daily quota. Women of childbearing years should get 400 micrograms of folic acid every day.

Like all moms (and doting aunts!), our hearts always dropped when Tammy's toddlers would take spills, fearing an injury. But we could rest assured knowing Tammy got her vitamin A and beta-carotene from her food when she was pregnant to help with the babies' bones and teeth development. Again, asparagus is your veggie to ensure that your baby has a good start as a toddler who won't break a bone every time he or she falls down. You'll get a hefty dose, nearly 13 percent of your daily need, just by sprinkling your salad with a cup of chopped raw asparagus.

Nothing creates a baby with a strong immune system that will easily fend off colds and flus like our Baby Bellas and Asparagus! As you appreciate their flavor, you can take pleasure in knowing

fortunate that the worst of her nausea lasted only a few weeks, during this time the only vegetable that appealed to her was asparagus, and so she loaded up on it as much as she could. Luckily, despite the morning sickness she was able to enjoy it many ways—steamed, grilled, roasted, with almonds, and in her Floating Asparagus Rafts, a way she liked to they'll help to do this thanks to asparagus's vitamin C. The vitamin C will also protect your baby's tissues from damage while helping absorb anemia-preventing iron. And asparagus is packed with that too! Iron is a mineral that is essential in the production of hemoglobin, the oxygen-carrying protein in red blood cells. Indulging in our Heavenly Roasted Vegetables will help prevent anemia, low birth weight, and premature delivery.

Next on the pregnancy checklist: B vitamins. Asparagus has bragging rights here! It contains nearly all of them, including riboflavin, thiamin, niacin, vitamin B_6, and of course folic acid. These provide a power-packed punch responsible for raising both your energy level and your baby's and maintaining it, helping with eyesight and healthy skin, nerves, and digestion. If you've got morning sickness, vitamin B_6 can help you with that, so grab a spear.

Asparagus even helps your body form muscles as well as red blood cells by providing vitamin E, a nutrient that most veggies fall short in. Pregnant? Keep any one of our asparagus dishes on the top shelf of your fridge at all times. This will also give you a dose of calcium. Thirty-two milligrams of calcium per cup isn't shabby for a veggie source of the bone-building mineral.

To ease the discomfort of pregnancy, asparagus is a must. Aside from the discomfort of a growing belly and adjusting to a shift in the center of gravity, constipation is all too common. With nearly 4 grams of fiber per cup of steamed asparagus, it's just the thing to keep you feeling good.

Asparagus beyond Pregnancy

Asparagus is a potent anti-inflammatory thanks to its saponins, one of which appears to play a role in preventing the inflammation from Lou Gehrig's disease. It also is one of the few vegetables that contains inulin and helps with digestive support. Additionally, asparagus helps with heart health, blood sugar regulation, and cancer prevention.

> **Some doctors suggest boosting folic acid intake from 400 to at least 600 micrograms daily once you're pregnant.**

Spotlight on Romaine Lettuce

Recipes with Romaine: Colorful Crunch Salad with Honey Dijon Vinaigrette, page 169; Herbed Romaine with Pine Nuts, page 176; Grab and Go Pita Slaw Sandwich, page 190

Our Mom always stacked our sandwiches with lettuce and tomatoes, but when Tammy was pregnant she took the word "stacked" to a whole new level when it came to romaine lettuce. No matter what her sandwich was made of—hummus, cheese, tuna, chicken, turkey, or veggie burger—she would pile on the lettuce so thick that it was a struggle to get her mouth around the sandwich. She liked it that way. She enjoyed the sweet flavor and fabulous crunch that the lettuce added and knowing she was doing something good for her health (and her twin babies') with every bite.

Romaine lettuce has endless health benefits, and it's stellar when it comes to pregnancy. Two cups of a romaine salad will give a pregnant woman more than 100 percent of her daily requirement for vitamin A and reassure her that she is doing her baby's bones and teeth good by helping them to grow. With every bite of lettuce providing a hefty dose of vitamin C, you can feel good knowing you're benefiting you and your baby. The lettuce is boosting your immunity, as well as your baby's, and helping with collagen formation and protecting cells from damage so you both can have healthy skin and tissues.

Enjoy two cups of our Herbed Romaine with Pine Nuts (page 176) daily and you'll be well on your way to fighting neural tube defects and spina bifida. From the lettuce alone, you'll get more than 13 percent of the folate that your pregnant body requires. And if you haven't already, you'll likely feel your baby start kicking! That's because romaine will also get you other B vitamins like thiamin, riboflavin, and vitamin B_6, which are important for giving you the energy that you need during your pregnancy. There's nothing like the exhaustion that pregnant women often feel, and these nutrients make romaine lettuce quite the

fatigue fighter while also helping to get your baby its energy and develop your baby's healthy skin, eyes, and nerves.

Have you ever wondered why romaine lettuce requires you to chew it several times before you can swallow it? That's thanks to its fiber. The fiber in lettuce also makes it desirable during pregnancy, as it helps to move wastes out quickly, reducing toxins in the body (you certainly don't want those lingering near your baby!) and keeping you regular and comfortable. If you stack your sandwich with about three leaves of lettuce, you'll get nearly an extra 2 grams of fiber. Not bad, considering you're also filling up on something that is packed with nutrients and provides a tasty crunch.

Romaine lettuce also doesn't disappoint when it comes to iron. It's a very good source, with close to 1 milligram for two cups of salad. So keep eating that romaine lettuce, tomato, and bean burrito to prevent a premature delivery and a low-birth-weight baby. That very same romaine-lettuce-filled burrito will also help your baby develop strong bones, thanks to its calcium. Many veggies don't contain calcium, but leafy greens like romaine are an exception.

Let-tuce Enjoy All of Romaine's Health Benefits

The health benefits of romaine lettuce don't end at pregnancy. It's one of the best veggies to fight the nation's obesity problem. Nearly every grocery store in

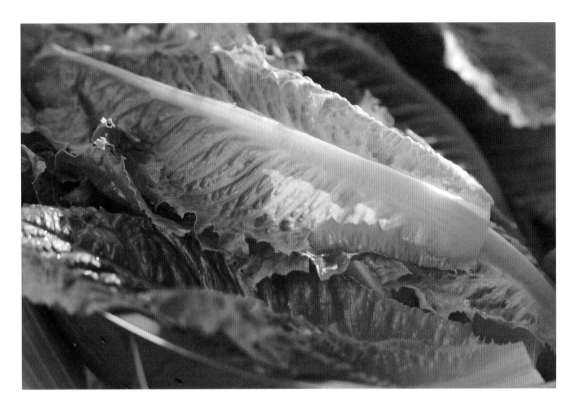

the country sells romaine, and it's the mainstay of a salad. Start your meal with a salad using a low-calorie dressing, like our Herbed Vinaigrette (page 184), Honey Dijon Vinaigrette (page 169), or plain balsamic vinegar, and research shows you'll eat fewer calories at your meal. The fiber in the romaine lettuce fills you up while providing very few calories. Plus, romaine is great for preventing heart attacks and strokes in more than one way, thanks to its vitamin C and beta-carotene that work in tandem by preventing cholesterol from sticking to artery walls. And thanks to the fiber in romaine lettuce, it also lowers cholesterol by dragging it out of the body.

Also contributing to a heart-healthy diet is romaine's folic acid and potassium content.

Beta-carotene is found in many fruits, grains, oils, and vegetables (green plants, carrots, sweet potatoes, squash, spinach, apricots, and green peppers) and becomes vitamin A in the small intestine. Vitamin A is mainly found in butter and eggs, so you should aim to get most of your vitamin A from beta-carotene, since fruits and vegetables are low in fat and are packed with vitamins and minerals, while butter is high in artery-clogging saturated fats.

CHAPTER 10

I Don't Have Time

Veggies for When You've Only Got Five Minutes

The Problem: You're crunched for time. You know veggies help keep you healthy and slim, and you want to eat them more often, but your hectic schedule often causes you to give veggies the shaft.

Here's What You Need: Frozen, canned, and pre-chopped veggies that can be whipped into a yummy veggie recipe packed with flavor and nutrients. Fresh or frozen pre-chopped cauliflower and broccoli florets, fresh or frozen stir-fry veggies, bagged cabbage and broccoli slaws, bagged washed spinach and greens, canned pumpkin, and diced canned tomatoes are just a few of the many great options.

Here's Why: Frozen veggies are just as nutritious as fresh ones, and you don't have to worry about them going bad. A selection of veggies in a well-stocked freezer ensures you can always prepare a healthful meal in a dash. With our easy-to-prepare tasty tricks, many canned veggies can be as healthful (or almost as healthful) and give you the benefits you desperately need and the flavor and texture you crave. Worrying about prep time will be a thing of the past. Veggies that are pre-chopped, washed-and-bagged,

canned, and frozen can be whipped into a delicious side in minutes or can be tossed in any meal—even when you order in!

The great thing about stovetop and microwave vegetable steaming is that it is fast and easy. It's a gentle heating method, so it allows vegetables to retain more of their color, texture, flavor, and nutrition.

> Try this delicious, nutrient-retaining, quick-cook option: Store low-sodium broth (our Vegetable Broth, page 164, or a store-bought variety; see chapter 17) in ice cube trays. Place a few frozen cubes in a sauté pan, heat them, add your veggies, and simmer for a couple of minutes. Voilà, you have a healthy and delish "sauté"!

Spotlight on Cauliflower

Recipes with Cauliflower: Cauliflower and Broccoli Flapjacks, page 115; Cauliflower Ceviche, page 127; Cauliflower Crusted Mozzarella Pie, page 186; Cream of Whatever Soup, page 159; Slam, Bam, Thank You Ma'am 5-Minute Broccoli or Cauliflower, page 235; The Nutrition Twins' Skinny Cauliflower Mash, page 238

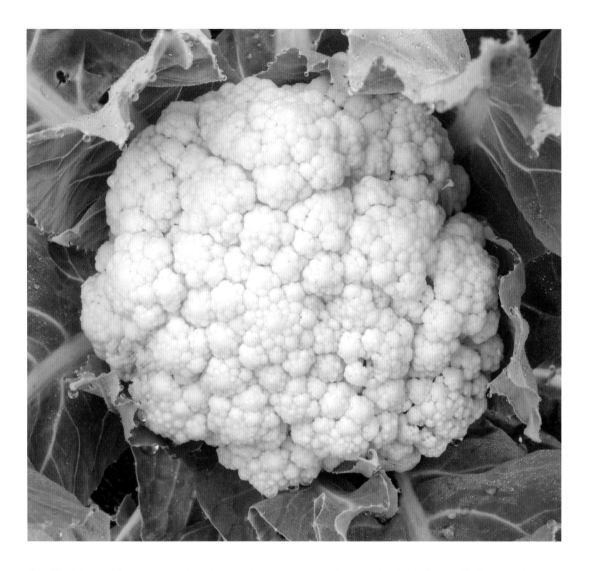

As dietitians it's no surprise that we have favorite cauliflower moments when we serve picky, non-veggie-eating kids (or entire families!) our version of mashed potatoes. We substitute cauliflower for the potatoes—"cauli-potatoes"—and it tastes just like the real deal. In fact, our tasters always devour our 30-calorie version without realizing that we swapped out the spuds. The bonus? Our recipe saves them more than 250 calories compared to a serving of the typical mashed potato recipe. If only they knew just how quickly we had prepared the dish.

If you need veggies in a hurry, you can find cauliflower in nearly all ready-to-go varieties—by the head, washed, bagged as florets, chopped and frozen.

All of these wonderful options make cauliflower consumption easy, no matter how hectic your life may be. Serve fresh precut cauliflower florets with hummus or dip on the dinner table. No prep necessary. Plus, it's endlessly adaptable, so within just minutes you can transform this perfect crudité into a pan-roasted cauliflower with garlic, lemon, and Parmesan or a cauliflower-enhanced pasta or soup, mashed "cauli-potatoes," cauliflower ceviche, or even cauliflower-crust pizza (see our Cauliflower Crusted Mozzarella Pie). Or simply toss pre-chopped cauliflower in a pan on the stove, and in minutes the cauliflower starts to brown and takes on a deep, nutty flavor. Add a little pepper, lemon, and garlic, and call it a delicious night. Ditto for the frozen variety.

Another way to serve up cauliflower in minutes? Steam it. Cauliflower steams on the stovetop in five minutes and in the microwave in three to four minutes. Then add our toppings (for suggestions see our Slam, Bam, Thank You Ma'am 5-Minute Broccoli or Cauliflower).

More cauliflower cooked in a jiffy? Heat five tablespoons of water or low-sodium broth in a skillet until it bubbles, add cauliflower florets, cover for five minutes, and voilà, you've got a great veggie to top with cheese or dressing, or to mash. Its texture is so versatile that you could puree it and add it to any soup (even canned) or casserole to make a tasty, more nutritiously delightful dish!

One hundred calories of cauliflower will give you a whopping 12 grams of fiber. Bye-bye constipation and bloat. And cauliflower is a member of the nutrient-packed cruciferous family that includes other nutritional rock stars like broccoli, brussels sprouts, cabbage, bok choy, and kale. This family is known for helping fight cancer because of its anti-inflammatory, antioxidant, and detoxifying nutrients. Cauliflower is loaded with phytonutrients like immune-boosting vitamin C and bone-healthy manganese and vitamin K. Plus, cauliflower is a great way to get folate, vitamin B_5, phosphorus, potassium, and magnesium. The last two will work to help relieve your body from the stress of your fast-paced lifestyle. Add cauliflower's power to fight heart disease and ward off or ease inflammation-related health problems like Crohn's disease, inflammatory bowel disease, insulin resistance, irritable bowel syndrome, metabolic syndrome, obesity, rheumatoid arthritis, type 2 diabetes, and ulcerative colitis, and you've got yourself one sweet deal that can be made in a dash.

Spotlight on Spinach

Recipes with spinach (17 of our recipes feature spinach; here's a handful): Berry Yogurt Detox Smoothie, page 106; Creamy Spinach Dip, page 134; Easy Spinach Pomodoro, page 214; Fruity Green Smoothie, page 108; Green Minted Cocoa Detox Smoothie; page 110; Minted Mango Melon Detox Smoothie, page 111; Roasted Red Pepper, Spinach, and Feta Portobello Burger, page 196; Spinach Squares, page 154; Veggie Yard Dash Salad, page 183

When we were growing up, our mom had two sure-fire hit dishes that she would make when she entertained. One was her spinach lasagna and the other was her meat lasagna. The spinach one was our favorite, and we'd often help her make it. When we went to college, we'd crave Mom's lasagna but didn't have the time to make it. So we invented our own version that took all of five minutes to prepare. We'd simply heat frozen spinach in a pot (often we'd let it defrost overnight in the fridge), then add our favorite low-sodium marinara sauce, lots of basil and oregano, and a sprinkle of pepper and low-fat mozzarella cheese. Lastly, we'd top it with a teaspoon of grated Parmesan. It was heaven! This dish was something we could really sink our teeth into (and whip up easily in a dorm room!), and we made it several times a week. We always felt good about eating it—we'd get lots of nutrients while enjoying a no-fuss dish.

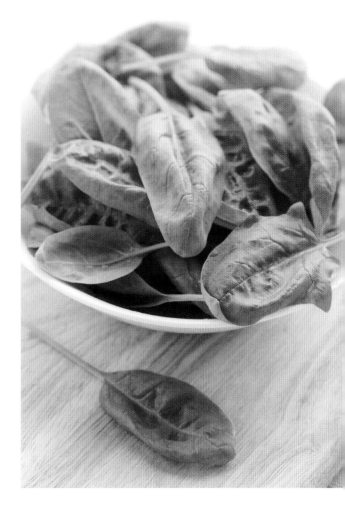

When you're in a rush, it's fantastic to know you can find spinach washed and bagged, frozen, and canned. At a moment's notice you can have the base of a salad, a delicious green as part of a wrap or to stuff in your sandwiches or as a side dish (Herb and Garlic Creamed Spinach, page 220), or a wonderful flavor and texture to add to a soup or stew (ciao, Herbed Pea Soup with Spinach, page 165)! Want pasta? Coarsely chop spinach leaves and toss them into a cold pasta salad or a hot pasta dish; the heat from the pasta is just enough to slightly wilt the leaves. Drinking a green smoothie? Include spinach for the perfect, invigoratingly fresh flavor. We promise—you won't even taste the greens!

Spinach leaves add color, texture, and bulk and a quick nutrient surge to any meal without contributing a lot of calories. For a speedy side dish you can quickly sauté an entire bag of spinach (frozen too) in a dab of oil and season—see our Simple Sautéed Spinach (page 234). And you can use this sauté as the base of many recipes, replacing some or all of the rice or noodles in a stir-fry. This will actually *save* you time, not to mention calories, while packing nutrients and fiber. Spinach makes it impossible to have an excuse to not have a veggie with dinner.

If your veggie consumption is limited, spinach is the perfect addition. It's super-nutrient-packed, and it boasts powerful antioxidant protection. It contains a range of phytonutrients like carotenoids, as well as flavonoids, and is an excellent source of other antioxidant nutrients including vitamin C, vitamin E, beta-carotene, manganese, zinc, and selenium. Spinach will also lift your vitality, thanks to iron and vitamin B_2, which will help convert food into energy. Plus, if you want to fight constipation, look no further: Spinach is a fantastic source of dietary fiber. You'll boost your bone health with vitamin K, magnesium, manganese, and calcium. You'll protect your heart with folate, potassium, and vitamin B_6.

Spinach packs a double protective punch for your heart and bones, as it not only contains the traditional nutrients mentioned above but also helps to combat oxidative-stress-related problems of the heart (clogged arteries and high blood pressure) and bones with its unusual combination of phytonutrients. If you want to be that girl or guy with glowing skin, healthy eyes, a strong skeleton, and a powerful immune system, eat no further than spinach. Is that our Fruity Green Smoothie we hear you blending up?

Spinach for the Eyes!

Did you know that 80 percent of visual impairment is avoidable? This includes macular degeneration. Simply get more lutein in your diet—it's found in dark greens, especially in spinach—and is an eye health powerhouse. To keep your eyes healthy, aim for 6 milligrams of lutein daily (most Americans get 1). The key is to go for cooked greens. In the raw form there are only about 2 milligrams of lutein in a cup of kale or spinach, but when cooked, spinach has 23 and kale 11. Lutein is most important during pregnancy for the development of the fetus's eyes. In addition, breast milk gets needed lutein to the baby after birth. Go for our Easy Spinach Pomodoro!

Although we don't recommend boiling most veggies, spinach is one of the exceptions. Simply boil it for one minute and discard the water. This will unbind oxalic acids and release them into the water, allowing the calcium found in spinach to be better absorbed. Added bonus? The spinach will taste sweeter.

CHAPTER 11

Mood-Boosting Must-Haves

Veggies That Lift Your Spirit

The Problem: You want that glowing, happy smile that makes people gravitate toward you. But you're tired and irritable, and smiling feels like work. You want life to feel more lighthearted and fun. You need a mood boost.

Here's What You Need: Your Happy Meal: a mood-boosting combination of omega-3 fats, vitamin E, vitamin D, selenium, vitamin B_6, vitamin C, folate, and high-fiber carbohydrates like those found in whole grains, fruits, and veggies. (We'll focus on the veggies to boost your mood here.)

Here's Why: While carbohydrates typically get an unfair shake these days, the ones found in vegetables boost serotonin, the body's feel-good chemical. Without it, your body's chemistry will be off and you'll be craving a mood boost. Folic acid, vitamin C, vitamin B_6, and vitamin E are all needed for your body to produce serotonin. People who are low in either vitamin D or omega-3 fatty acids have higher rates of depression. Omega-3 fats appear to boost mood for people with mild depression.

Here's How to Get It: Indulging in a piece of chocolate cake may be what comes to mind when you want to lift your spirits, but that will only leave you craving another mood boost and more sweet treats after the sugar crash. Try these long-lasting mood boosters instead:

• **Go for quality carbohydrates.** The serotonin created by the vegetables that are higher in carbs will help to soothe you and lift your mood. Some of the best-quality carbohydrates come from vegetables, because they are low in calories and fat and offer other mood-lifting nutrients. Think potatoes, butternut squash, spaghetti squash, peas, and corn.

• **Go for vitamin E from leafy greens** like spinach and turnip greens, and from bell peppers, broccoli, and asparagus.

• **To feel "D"-lighted, eat mushrooms.** Portobello and crimini are among the highest in vitamin D, but all mushrooms are good sources. Mushrooms are the only vegetable that contain vitamin D, and some are grown with special lights, so a serving can offer your entire daily requirements for this happy vitamin. Without adequate vitamin D, you're more likely to feel sad.

• **To avoid feeling blue, go for the greens.** You'll get folic acid from salad greens like spinach and romaine lettuce, as well as from beans, green peas, mushrooms, asparagus, eggplant, corn, carrots, and cruciferous vegetables such as cauliflower and broccoli.

• **B happy! Get your quota of vitamin B$_6$** with summer squash, bell peppers, turnip greens, shiitake mushrooms, spinach, garlic, cauliflower, mustard greens, cabbage, crimini mushrooms, asparagus, broccoli, kale, collard greens, and brussels sprouts.

• **To be Cheerful, Chipper, and Content, get your vitamin C.** Bell peppers, broccoli, tomatoes, kale, cauliflower, and potatoes are all sources.

Spotlight on Sweet Potatoes

Recipes with Sweet Potatoes: Coco Sweet Potatoes with Mango Salsa, page 130; Chipotle Smashed Sweet Potatoes, page 212; Curried Sweet Potato and Apple Salad, page 132; Savory Sweet Potato Fries, page 153; Sweet Potato Veggie Burgers, page 203

Some of our favorite childhood memories include family mealtimes centered on our mom's home cooking. Sitting down to Mom's food always made us happy—it was soothing and lifted our spirits if we were ever upset. We each have memories of sitting at the table and enjoying one of our favorite comfort foods: sweet potatoes. Whether they were mashed, baked, grilled, broiled, or simply in a soup, smoothie, salad, or latkes, we loved every variety of this home-cooked comfort food. From their sweet, creamy, and flavorful center to their crunchy and robust skin, they made us feel satisfied and content. It always seemed like there was nothing a sweet potato couldn't make better. And now we know why.

If you've got the blues, sweet potatoes are just the medicine you need to lift your spirits. They're one of the best, most nutritious sources of carbohydrates. And carbohydrates are your happy bite when it comes to feeling content and at your best. When you consume carbohydrates, they create a surge in endorphins like serotonin, chemicals that lift mood. They make you feel good and it shows; people are attracted to positivity and want to be around you. But without carbohydrates, brain chemistry will go awry and favor depression. In fact, not only do people with low levels of serotonin show signs of depression, but they are more anxious, they don't sleep as well, and they are moodier. The carbohydrates in sweet potatoes come with fiber and loads of phytonutrients in a virtually fat-free package—as long as you avoid those high-calorie toppings!

The moment our clients hear that they can eat a sweet potato, they light up. That's because sweet potatoes are not only delicious but also satisfying, and when people come to see a nutritionist, they always think it means that they'll soon feel deprived. Try this test: Serve Savory Sweet Potato Fries or our Chipotle Smashed Sweet Potatoes to someone you love and tell them how good sweet potatoes are for them (this doesn't include french fried sweet potatoes—or those loaded with butter, maple syrup, and marshmallows!) and watch the response. Your loved one will be rewarded with a tasty meal, and you get the benefit of seeing them satiated and uplifted.

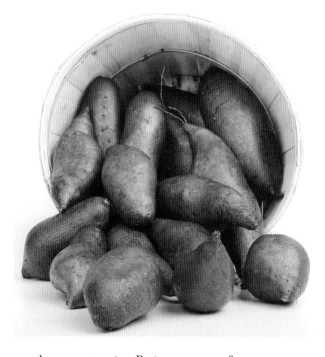

Eating sweet potatoes don't cause your energy to come crashing down as many other carbohydrates do. The fiber in the potato causes the glucose from the carbohydrates to enter your bloodstream at a more gradual rate, helping to keep your energy level stable and aiding in the prevention of mood swings that come with energy highs and lows. The fiber also allows for a longer, more sustained serotonin surge. One small sweet potato contains nearly 4 grams of fiber, and the fiber in sweet potatoes keeps you regular, light, and happy. Thank you, fiber!

Sweet potatoes are a rich source of vitamin B_6, another vitamin necessary to keep spirits high. One cup baked contains 17 percent of the daily value for this important nutrient. Like carbohydrates, vitamin B_6 is required to produce serotonin. B_6 is necessary for the creation of amines, a type of messaging molecule or neurotransmitter that the nervous system relies on to send signals from one nerve to the next. If you don't have enough vitamin B_6, amines can't be created and neither can serotonin. The happy chain will never even begin. Plus, without B_6, melatonin, the hormone needed for a good night's rest, can't be created either. Sleep rejuvenates serotonin. So if you don't have enough B_6, you won't be able to get the sleep your body needs to function at its peak. Not only will you feel fatigued, but you'll also be uncomfortable and unhappy. Prevent this from happening by indulging in a sweet potato. And just hearing that you can and should eat a sweet potato will boost your mood. It's a happy cycle!

The bliss created by sweet potatoes doesn't end there. They're an excellent source of vitamin C, with a cup of baked sweet potato providing 37.2 percent of the vitamin C you need in a day. Vitamin C is best known for its powerful antioxidant properties, which will make you feel good by helping your body to produce your happy hormone serotonin. And vitamin C boosts your immunity, keeping you healthy so that you can enjoy feeling good.Vitamin C is also needed to produce neurotransmitters like dopamine, the chemical that gives you that feel-good high that you get when you're in love. Dopamine helps us deal with stress and relax. People with a vitamin C deficiency often feel fatigued or depressed. Additionally, vitamin C enhances the absorption of energy-boosting iron, also making vitamin C essential for overcoming stress and maintaining a healthy brain. Sweet potatoes do for your mood what a face-lift does for your face. And as an extra bonus, when you smile and exude happiness, you look like you got a face-lift anyway!

Sweeeeet! Potato

Sweet potatoes are superstars when it comes to a mood lift, but their benefits don't end there. They contain two very potent antioxidants—carotenoids and sporamins, which fight everything from the negative health consequences that come with aging to almost all types of disease. Additionally, sweet potatoes are true superheroes when it comes to fighting inflammation. Research shows that when you eat a sweet potato, inflammation in the body immediately decreases, especially in the brain and nerve tissues throughout the body. When it comes to type 2 diabetes, sweet potatoes also seem to offer great promise. Lastly, more new research shows sweet potatoes' glycosides have strong antibacterial and antifungal properties, and as we eat our Sweet Potato Veggie Burger, we look forward to what will be discovered.

Want a sports edge? Eat a sweet potato. Aside from providing long-lasting energy from carbohydrates that are packed with fiber, sweet potatoes are loaded with vitamin B_6. This vitamin is necessary for the breakdown of glycogen, the form in which sugar is stored in muscles and the liver, so vitamin B_6 is critical when it comes to athletic performance and endurance.

Spotlight on Spaghetti Squash

Recipes with Spaghetti Squash: Spaghetti Squash with Fresh Tomato Sauce, page 200

Over the years we've had countless people tell us that they love pasta but stay away from it because it makes them gain weight. They miss their comfort food and simply wish that they could devour a

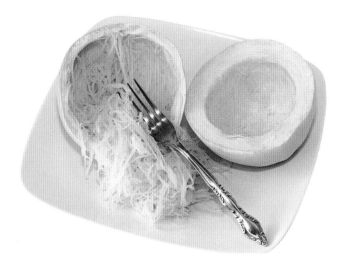

bowl of angel hair without feeling guilty about what it was doing to their waistline.

Do you wish you could eat your comfort food without guilt? Guess what? You can! Enter spaghetti squash. We were first introduced to spaghetti squash in our adult years when our friend Joan raved about it, telling us how easy it was to prepare the "spaghetti" in the microwave. She would cook it until soft, shred it into "pasta" with a fork, then add a little tomato sauce, a sprinkle of Parmesan, and voilà, she had a low-calorie variety of her beloved comfort food. It was her favorite dinner, and every time she ate it she'd feel so satisfied. It also turns out that her delicious pasta alternative was saving her 170 calories per baked cup compared to whole wheat spaghetti.

Spaghetti squash, like most winter squash, is one of the vegetables highest in carbohydrates. Just as the carbohydrates in sweet potatoes boost mood, so do the carbohydrates in winter squash; they combat pain and create a mental

calmness and serenity. Remember, carbohydrates are a necessity when it comes to boosting endorphins like serotonin. Boost those endorphins, and immediately you'll feel like you're on cloud nine. So it's a real happy pill. And the carbohydrates in spaghetti squash are very different from the "feared" ones that you find in refined pasta, because the squash version comes packed with fiber and nutrients and less than a third of the carbohydrates that you'd find in a cup of regular pasta. The fiber promotes gradual digestion and a steady supply of energy, extending the happy boost and creating a long-lived mood surge that will allow you to stay on your cloud. An added bonus of endorphins? They decrease appetite.

Aside from carbohydrates, spaghetti squash also contains specific nutrients needed to turn the tryptophan in certain foods into serotonin. Without these nutrients and without serotonin, your mood will suffer, and so will every aspect of your life; when you don't feel content, even the best things in life are less appealing. Spaghetti squash is a good source of folic acid, vitamin B_6, and vitamin C, all of which are responsible for turning tryptophan into serotonin. One cup of the baked uplifting veggie contains 17 percent of the daily requirement of vitamin B_6, more than 10 percent of the daily value for folic acid, and 9 percent of the daily value for vitamin C. And guess what? Spaghetti squash contains tryptophan. So it doesn't just turn other foods into a feel-good food, it turns itself into a fun house, a real party extravaganza.

Spaghetti squash's mood-enhancing powers don't end there. Research has found that people who suffer from depression often have low blood levels of omega-3 fatty acids. Spaghetti squash is one of the few vegetables that contain a small amount of omega-3 fats. One cup of baked squash provides 121 milligrams of omega-3s in the form of alpha-linolenic acid (ALA).

Additionally, spaghetti squash is a good source of magnesium. Magnesium has a calming effect that relaxes the body and makes you feel good. Plus, spaghetti squash has potassium, which helps dilate your blood vessels, lowering your blood pressure and taking the edge off, thereby providing a further calming effect. All of these attributes make spaghetti squash a real tension-tamer, which will give a boost to even the most anxiety-ridden. It's a true upper.

Other Reasons You'll Get a Kick (and a Smile) out of Spaghetti Squash

Spaghetti squash, like other winter squash and members of the *Cucurbita* genus, is an antioxidant powerhouse. Aside from the vitamin C and the antioxidant mineral manganese, spaghetti squash also contains phenolic phytonutrients, which help to prevent damage to our cells, reduce the risk of disease, and hinder the aging process. Who doesn't want to enjoy spaghetti *and* the benefits of a body that functions the way it did when it was younger?

And like other winter squash, spaghetti squash has long been recognized for its health-promoting alpha-carotene and beta-carotene, lutein, zeaxanthin, and beta-cryptoxanthin. These carotenoids are important for everything from protecting against cancer to helping to prevent macular degeneration. Spaghetti squash also functions as a powerful anti-inflammatory that helps to protect against disease, thanks to the pectin in the cell walls of the squash.

Lastly, spaghetti squash helps with blood sugar regulation, so if you are at risk for diabetes or it runs in your family, trade in your refined, insulin-spiking pasta for some spaghetti squash.

Want a crunchy snack? Spaghetti squash seeds can be roasted just like pumpkin seeds (after all, pumpkin is a squash). They are nutritious, and delicious!

What's the easiest way to cook spaghetti squash? Rinse the skin. Pierce it several times with a sharp knife. Do this especially if you're microwaving it, or you may end up with a "squash explosion." Then you can do what we do: Toss it in the microwave for 10 to 12 minutes and then let it stand for 5 minutes to finish steaming. Just know it will be very hot when you cut it open. Prefer to bake it? Put it in the oven for about an hour at 375°F.

CHAPTER 12

Hunger Games

Veggies You Can Sink Your Teeth Into

The Problem: You're hungry. You arrive at meals feeling ravenous and end up overeating the wrong foods—and then you suffer the consequences, feeling stuffed, bloated, and lousy.

Here's What You Need: Veggies, particularly ones that you can sink your teeth into, with a "meaty" feel, like eggplant, all mushrooms, beans, potatoes, pumpkin, winter squash, parsnips, carrots, and steamed cabbage and greens. These fill you up and are satisfying but leave you feeling content, light, and comfortable rather than stuffed and puffy.

Here's Why: Chewing satisfaction begins in the mouth, and the texture of veggies like eggplant and mushrooms imitates the sensation of biting into a texture-rich protein. The fiber in the veggies will fill your stomach with substance, making you satiated and content. Plus, the more a food weighs, the more it will fill you. Think volume. Water is heavy, and most vegetables are 80 to 95 percent water, so they fill you up without any extra calories (gotta love this!).

Raw leafy greens and cabbage won't fill your stomach the way their steamed/cooked variety will. When raw, they are light and airy and won't be as satisfying. When you steam them (even in the microwave) they become more compact and voluminous.

Spotlight on Eggplant

Recipes with Eggplant: Eggplant Parmesan, page 187; Mediterranean Pizza, page 192; Rockin' Ratatouille, page 152

Interestingly, when we ask our meat-loving clients to name some of their favorite restaurant meals, among the meat dishes they typically include eggplant Parmesan. If you've ever eaten eggplant Parmesan, this probably comes as no surprise, as you're well aware that this purple veggie has a meaty, solid texture, spongy and satisfying to bite—one reason that makes it an ideal stand-in for the meat in chicken or veal Parmesan or many other favorite Italian dishes.

Ever have a day when you feel like your appetite is insatiable? A day when you could easily consume thousands of calories in an attempt to satisfy your hunger and then still want more? Are you looking for something that you can sink your teeth into but that won't leave you with a waistline that your finger sinks into for inches? Look no further than eggplant, the perfect answer and the ideal alternative to calorie-packed disasters. With a hearty texture and

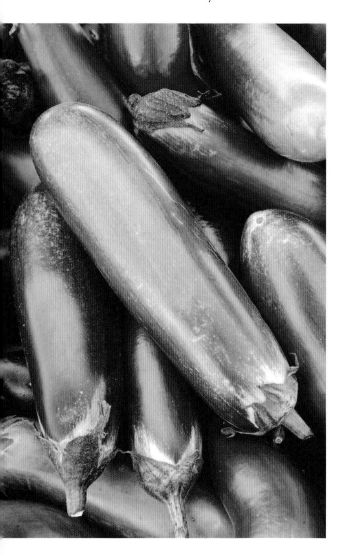

delicious flavor, eggplant has a mere 35 calories in an entire cooked cup. It's no wonder eggplant is commonly used to replace meat in lasagnas and pastas or as a substitute for chicken in chicken Parmesan. It gives your mouth the texture and flavor you crave and your stomach the substance it desires, thanks to its high volume. High-volume foods have a high water and fiber content, and eggplant is loaded with both. Eat high-volume foods and you'll leave each meal feeling satisfied, but you won't be eating a lot of extra calories. You'll fill yourself up but not out! Eggplant will satisfy your seemingly unquenchable hunger. Try our Eggplant Parmesan, Mediterranean Pizza, or Rockin' Ratatouille and you'll never turn to other calorie-dense, waist-line-sabotaging foods again.

Another great thing about eggplant is its nutrition value. In addition to its fiber, some of which is soluble (the kind that helps lower blood cholesterol levels), eggplant is loaded with antioxidants, like immune-boosting vitamin C, B vitamins, and heart-healthy potassium. Eggplant has bone-building nutrients—vitamin K, manganese, and magnesium. Most people don't get enough purple-colored veggies, and the deep purple skin of the eggplant contains anthocyanins and proanthocyanins, antioxidants that may aid heart health and improve brain function. Eggplant also boasts chloro-genic acid, one of the most powerful free radical scavengers in plants, which helps fight cancer, provides antimicrobial and antiviral benefits, and helps lower "bad" LDL cholesterol.

Eggplant's spongy texture soaks up oil quickly, so to keep it lean, avoid cooking methods that include frying or sautéing. You can also help the eggplant absorb less oil if you "sweat" it. You may have seen eggplant recipes that have you sweat the eggplant by salting it. This is often recommended to make its texture more tender and to lessen some of its naturally occurring bitterness. After slicing the eggplant, sprinkle it with salt and let it sit for about a half hour. This will pull out some of its water content and make it less absorptive of any oil used in cooking. Just be sure to rinse the eggplant after sweating, which will remove most of the salt.

Spotlight on Portobello Mushrooms

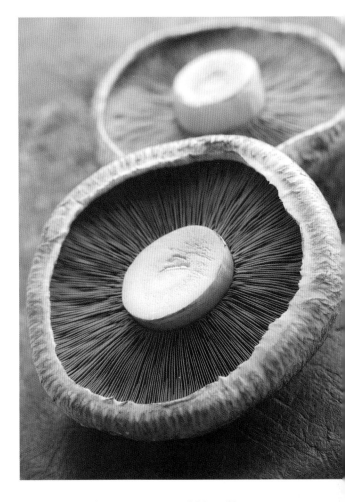

Recipes with Portobello Mushrooms: Baby Bellas and Asparagus, page 206; Hot Diggity Chili!, page 195; Italian Mushrooms, Tomato, and Spinach, page 224; Roasted Red Pepper, Spinach, and Feta Portobello Burger, page 196; Stuffed Peppers, page 202

The first time we ate portobello mushrooms was as teenagers when we joined our parents at their friend's house for a barbecue. We had just started to embrace our healthy lifestyle, and when asked if we'd like a burger or "veggie" burger, we were intrigued by the veggie one. When we sunk our teeth into our portobello mushroom burgers, we could hardly believe the juicy, rich flavor and meaty texture weren't coming from meat. Our taste buds fell in love. And when we finished eating and felt content and satiated, yet light and energetic, unlike the sluggish feelings we had after eating meat burgers, we never looked at meat—or at mushrooms—the same way again.

Do you often find yourself arriving at meals overly hungry and then overeating heavy, meaty foods, thinking they're the only things that will fill you up? Often find yourself digging your hearty appetite into something meaty to put a lid on your cravings? If you have a relentless appetite, portobello mushrooms are an unbelievable find. Thick and juicy with their meaty texture, they seem just as tender and delicious as a real cut of beef. The ultimate MLV. Yes, a Meat Lover's Vegetable that is often larger than six inches in diameter and makes a phenomenal substitute for beefsteaks and other types of grilled meat (also great stuffed). Throw them on the grill, add some seasoning, and voilà—you'll get the same smoky and flavorful taste as an actual steak.

You could devour a beef quarter-pounder for 320 calories and get nearly half of your daily allotment for artery-clogging fat plus the undesirable after-bloat. But why would you want to do that when you can sink your teeth into a quarter-pound Roasted Red Pepper, Spinach, and Feta Portobello Burger for 53 calories? The portobello variety also has no artery-clogging fat or cholesterol, and you get one-sixth the calories that you'd find in the beef.

In fact, if you ate 320 calories of portobello burgers (not that you need to eat this many—one or two should suffice, although they're so delicious you might want to devour even more!), you'd also get more than 24 grams of fiber (there's none in beef), which is less than 1 gram

shy of your entire daily quota! No wonder the portobellos are so satisfying: That fiber expands in your stomach, taking up space and filling you.

Another reason portobello mushrooms curb hunger? About 160 grams yields 45 percent protein; that's 4 grams of protein in 35 calories. So if you eat 320 calories' worth, you're consuming 36 grams of protein, which is more than the 29 grams you get in the beef variety! Go for the portobello and you fill your stomach and finally squash your hunger, but without the bloat and puffiness or the threat to your waistline.

Although you're surely already sold on portobellos, don't close their cap just yet, as portobellos not only satisfy your hunger, but they're also packed with phytonutrients that support the immune system and prevent inflammation—helping to protect against arthritis, cancer, and heart disease (see chapter 3). Portobellos (and white button too) provide traditional vitamins and minerals such as immune-boosting vitamin D, zinc, and selenium, and energy-producing B vitamins like pantothenic acid, niacin, and vitamin B_2, as well as heart-healthy potassium, folate, B_1, and B_6. Trace minerals iron, copper, and bone-healthy manganese are also what you sink your teeth into with this next bite of our "Veggie Meat." Can't wait until you try our Baby Bellas and Asparagus!

CHAPTER 13

Detox and Cleanse

Veggies That Flush Toxins after Overindulgence

The Problem: You've overdone it and now you're hurting. You've got a hangover. Whether it's from too much alcohol, too much salt, or just plain overeating, you're paying the price. You feel tired, waterlogged, and heavy. You likely have a bloated belly, puffiness under your eyes, swollen hands and feet, and a headache. And you may be constipated to boot.

Here's What You Need: An immediate fix to bring an abrupt end to the symptoms and discomfort associated with overdoing it. You need . . . a veggie "detox." It will immediately get your body and mind back on the healthy track. Packed with anti-inflammatory compounds and antioxidants, potassium, and fiber, but low in calories and sodium, it'll hydrate you and give you a good cleanse. Veggies, blended into drinks and shakes, are the perfect remedy. And on days when you don't have time to turn them into drinks, at least be sure to go for any veggie that helps with the elimination and restoration process, or choose our Refreshing Beet and Watermelon Detox Salad (page 181) or our Cool Cucumber Bites (page 211), which also serve as a detox.

Here's Why: The last thing you want is something high in calories and heavy; it will only dig you further into a hole. Most veggies are 80 to 90 percent water—or more—and are good sources of potassium. Together these help your body to function properly and help to flush out salt or any other toxins. The veggies will flood your bloodstream with a high dose of antioxidant and anti-inflammatory nutrients to prevent invaders from damaging your body and help to rinse out destructive free radicals.

Your body extracts nutrients from the food you eat, and the leftovers go to your colon along with all of the other "garbage" your body doesn't use. Think of high-fiber veggies as a broom coming into your toxin-filled colon and sweeping your insides clean, swiftly shuttling toxins out of your body—the ultimate cleanse. Veggies will make you feel so much better that you'll almost think the "too much" never happened.

Here's How to Get It: You want all veggies that are packed with water, potassium, fiber, antioxidants, and anti-inflammatory compounds. This means almost all vegetables, although some are particularly high in these nutrients and also contain additional and special detox nutrients. Some of the vegetables highest in water content are lettuce, celery, cucumber, spinach, zucchini, and cabbage; some of the most potassium-packed veggies are kale, spinach, chard, mushrooms, zucchini, and asparagus. Broccoli, brussels sprouts, carrots, and cauliflower are among the ultimate veggies in terms of fiber; and beets, bok choy, fennel, and kale contain these plus additional detoxifying phytonutrients.

Spotlight on Beets

Recipes with Beets: Beet and Carrot Savory Pancakes, page 114; Refreshing Beet and Watermelon Detox Salad, page 181; Swiss Chard Salad with Red and Golden Beets and Honey Yogurt Vinaigrette, page 182

As kids we knew beets as borscht from a jar—a red beet soup served cold with a dollop of sour cream. Our grandma was from Russia's Ukraine, and although she made all meals from scratch, for some reason she started off dinner meals with this bottled borscht. Some people believe Russians live for a long time because they eat so much borscht. Admittedly, we skipped this course, as we were quite picky little kids and didn't like sour cream *or* borscht. It wasn't until we were adults that we got up the courage to try beets—and that was only after learning that they were nutrition rock stars. After all, we couldn't continue to boast about being adventurous with healthy foods if we didn't give raw beets a try. To our very pleasant surprise, beets weren't at all how we remembered them from the jarred soup. We enjoyed their sweet, rich, yet earthy flavor and thought they tasted somewhat like carrots. We're a fan of their crunch and how they add a wonderful sweetness to a green smoothie. In fact, at times we may even choose a beet over a carrot, and particularly on a day when we feel we just had *too much.*

Beets indeed are great for cleansing the body. Overdid it on Chinese food last night? Alcohol? Rich indulgences? This is not the time to beet shy. For starters, beets are a good source of fiber to sweep the toxins (like those from overindulging) from your colon. You'll get close to 4 grams of fiber—15 percent of what you need in an entire day—in just a cup of beets. Say au revoir to last night's fried pork dumplings! And beets' potassium will help restore fluid balance in your swelled body while flushing out the salt. Adios bloat and high blood pressure. And like all veggies, beets are a great way to get water to rinse your system. But beyond all of these purifying components, what truly makes beets a detoxification gold mine and sets them apart on the detox battlefield is their nutrient-packed punch from their phytonutrient pigments.

A prime champion in beets' detox support? Their betalain pigments. These pigments have special capabilities to activate our bodies' detox system; they ensure that toxic substances are

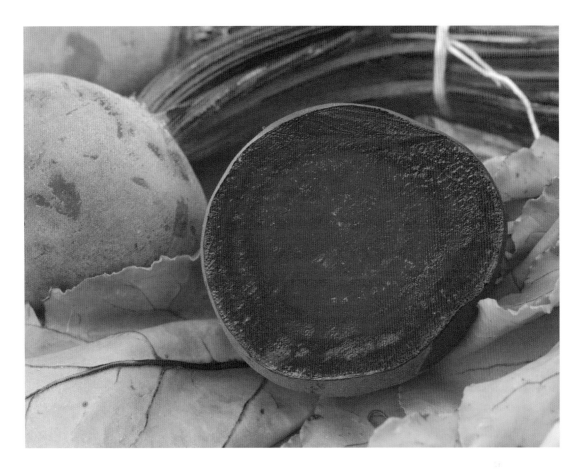

neutralized and made water-soluble so that we can excrete them in our urine. It doesn't end there. Beets trigger not just one detox system in our body but multiple pathways that are extremely critical in the detox process. And since the concentration of betalains in both the peel and the flesh of beets is high, eating beets makes an easy way to get a great cleanse. So even if you didn't have a night of overdoing it but are someone who thinks about exposure to toxins and wants to give your body as much detox support as possible, beets are for you.

Complementing their purifying power, beets have an enormous antioxidant and anti-inflammatory component to help prevent the toxins that enter our body from oxidizing and from causing inflammation and damage to the body. Remember, free radicals are destructive particles that enter our body simply from normal daily living, like breathing and stress—you don't even have to overdo it to have free radicals in your body!—and beets' antioxidants help to detoxify these. Beets have a very unusual mix of antioxidant phytonutrients that do this. While most red vegetables get their beautiful color from anthocyanins, beets get most of their color from betalain, which, as you now know, has major cleansing capability. In addition, betalain is a potent antioxidant. This means that in case its first attempts to purify your body by activating your detox pathways didn't work, it's got antioxidants that also squash toxins so that they can be excreted. Combine this with beets' powerful antioxidants vitamin C and manganese, and you have an incredible vegetable to crush and excrete foreign invaders.

And if your heart wasn't already beating faster for beets, there's more. Beets prevent inflammation. Chronic inflammation is linked to diabetes, heart disease, depression, and cancer. And beets help to fight these diseases beyond their anti-inflammatory powers, since they are packed with disease-fighting phytonutrients as well. Beets are a great source of fiber, and remarkably a large portion of their fiber comes from pectin, which is only found in a handful of other vegetables, like carrots and green beans. The fiber may provide special health benefits, especially in our digestive tract (including prevention of colon cancer) and our cardiovascular system. In addition to being high in water, fiber, and potassium, beets are an excellent source of heart-healthy folate and a very good source of the free-radical-squashing antioxidants manganese, vitamin C,

and copper; bone-helping magnesium; and iron and phosphorus to help boost energy. Just 10 more reasons to load up on beets. Beet and Carrot Savory Pancakes, anyone?

Handle These Powerful Purifiers with Care

Did you know that beets don't just come in a reddish-purple shade? They can have white, golden/yellow, and even rainbow-colored roots. No matter what their color, they aren't as tough as they look; the smallest bruise or break causes red beets' red-purple pigments (which contain a variety of phytonutrients including betalains and anthocyanins) to bleed, especially during cooking. Betalain pigments in beets are extremely water soluble, and they are also temperature sensitive. To retain the nutrients, treat beets as a delicate food, even though they might seem "rock solid" and difficult to damage.

Beets are a different variety within the same plant family (Amaranthaceae-Chenopodiaceae) as Swiss chard. The beet's green leaves, which connect to the root (the part we call the beet), have a similar and delicious taste and texture and can be prepared like Swiss chard or spinach. They are a nutrient powerhouse, concentrated in vitamins, minerals, and carotenoids like beta-carotene and lutein/zeaxanthin.

Raw beetroots have a crunchy texture that turns soft and buttery when they are cooked. Beet leaves have a lively, bitter taste similar to chard, so they can be versatile in recipes.

Spotlight on Kale

Recipes with Kale: Dieter's Delight Chock Full of Veggies Soup, page 163; Grapefruit, Avocado, and Kale Salad with Pepitas, page 174; Guilt-Free Kale Chips, page 143

We're always amused to think of our past when we were little girls who found it a chore to stop playing in the yard and come inside to eat dinner. That's because, somewhere along the way, we became those girls who get excited over a mouthwatering kale salad. Although we have appreciated good food and our veggies for years now, we believe that our love affair with kale began in a little restaurant on Manhattan's Lower East Side where we licked our plate clean after enjoying a kale salad with a little lemon and garlic and some steamed butternut squash. And now we're obsessed.

We're particularly enamored of curly red kale, but lacinato (also known as dinosaur kale) floats our boat too. It really shouldn't be a surprise, since kale is a member of the cabbage family, another love of ours. Once you learn about kale's role in detoxing and try our delicious Dieter's Delight Chock Full of Veggies Soup after a night of

overindulgence, prepare to have a love affair of your own. If you've seen kale in the market and been intimidated by it, fear no more, we'll show you kale's delicious detox side.

Have a food (or alcohol) hangover that's left you feeling regretfully bloated in the belly, puffy under the eyes, or with swollen fingers? Want to flush out the damage as fast as possible? Say hello to Prince Charming, kale. Like any knight in shining armor, kale's got a slew of defense tactics to keep your body pure. For starters, kale's got 2.6 grams of fiber in a cup—that's 7 grams of fiber in 100 calories' worth, all on standby to sweep out those leftover toxins from your overindulgence that are hanging out in your colon. Meanwhile, kale is 85 percent water and potassium packed, a brilliant combo to help to restore normal fluid balance while rinsing out bloating salt and flushing out other toxins as the body neutralizes them, preventing damage.

What really sets kale apart from the other suitors when it comes to cleansing your body is the specific role it has in supporting the body's detoxification processes. Most toxins that harm the body must be detoxified using our body's two-phase decontamination process. There is phase I detoxification and phase II detoxification, and kale helps with both. What's more, kale has a uniquely high amount of sulfur compounds—and it's these that are needed to support phase II detoxification. So if you had a bit too much to drink last night or if you

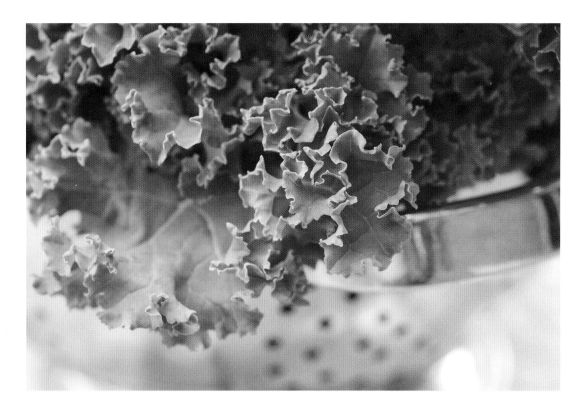

had a bit too much of anything, have our Grapefruit, Avocado, and Kale Salad with Pepitas. It will activate both stages of your body's detox system, and its nutrients will give your body a real advantage in counteracting toxic exposure, whether from your environment or from your food.

What makes kale the perfect catch is that it has so much to offer even aside from its detox capabilities. Kale is an ultimate nutritional all-star. It's packed with anti-inflammatory and antioxidant nutrients and has been linked to a reduction in oxidative stress and the health problems related to it, like cancer, cataracts, atherosclerosis, and chronic obstructive pulmonary disease (COPD). And kale's phytonutrients combat many of these diseases from a different angle, making kale a solid protector against chronic diseases. Kale is an outstanding source of bone-healthy vitamin K (one cup of kale provides far more than most other high sources). Plus, vitamin K is a key nutrient for helping regulate our body's inflammatory process. Kale is an excellent source of vitamins A and C and manganese, and it's a very good source of fiber, potassium, B_6, and calcium and a good source of omega-3 fats, magnesium, folate, iron, and vitamin E.

CHAPTER 14

Salad Haters' Delights

Veggies for Irresistible Bowl Creations

You do want to be healthy and look lean and fit, but you refuse to feel like a rabbit nibbling on a boring meal of lettuce leaves. And we don't blame you. You deserve to get the nutrients that you need *and* enjoy one of life's finest pleasures— eating. And a one- or two-vegetable salad drenched in dressing isn't going to cut it. In fact, it'll just leave you feeling hungry and deprived after swallowing more calories from the dressing than you'd get from a burger. Surprisingly, it's typically the people with the best intentions to eat "just" a salad for weight loss that end up falling off the diet wagon. Skimpy salads typically cause weight gain due to extreme hunger, which often leads to devouring excessive calories while trying to feel satisfied. If you're currently not a fan of salads for these very reasons, these tips are for you.

The great news is that you can truly create a mouthwatering, delectable salad that will not only leave you wanting to lick your bowl but will also help you to fight cravings and lose weight. The beneficial veggies in these salads fight chronic health conditions like heart disease, diabetes, cancer, and obesity—all in one bowl! The key is crafting a salad with pizazz, using a variety of flavors from earth's most prized possessions—sweet, zesty, savory—and a crunch that you can really sink your teeth into. Do this and immediately you'll have a winning combination.

The Problem: You think salads are boring, so you avoid them altogether or only eat them doused in dressing.

Here's What You Need: Salads with pizazz—crunchy or soft textures and/or unusual flavors.

Here's Why: Ninety-nine percent of salads contain the same vegetables—tomatoes, iceberg lettuce, and carrots. Salads need new flavors and textures to keep people interested and excited so they don't feel the need to rely on calorie-laden dressing for flavor. By avoiding the dressing pitfall and incorporating exciting superstar ingredients, you'll get even more nutrients without negating the positive health aspects of the salad.

Here's How to Get It: Add sparkle to your salad with the crunch and color of water chestnuts, artichoke hearts, snow peas, corn kernels, baby corn, string beans, and chopped asparagus—or add zest with roasted bell peppers and diced olives and fennel.

Spotlight on Corn

Recipes with Corn: Corn and Bean Salsa, page 131; Edamame and Corn Salad, page 173; Hot Diggity Chili!, page 195; Quinoa with Mixed Vegetables, page 193; Stuffed Peppers, page 202; Veggie Yard Dash Salad, page 183

Note: Although corn is widely classified as a grain and is typically included in research studies of whole grain foods like wheat, oats, and barley, the kernels that we call "corn" are technically the fruit of the *Zea mays* plant. Corn offers many similar benefits to veggies and a health-supportive combination of antioxidant phytonutrients, and in the United States most people (including us!) think of it as a veggie, so we include it here.

Whenever we ask our clients what vegetables they like, corn is invariably on their short list. And is it any wonder why? After all, corn is sweet and succulent, and there is nothing more satisfying then digging your teeth into an ear of fresh summer kernels. Even kids (and adults!) with the pickiest palates love corn's sweet flavor. When you think about summertime grilling in the backyard, no barbecue is complete without the fresh crunch of corn. Eating corn was especially fun for us because our dad taught us the secret to eating corn without getting any kernels (not even one!) stuck in our teeth, while also teaching us to remove every single kernel from the cob, mimicking machine-grade perfection. In the Lakatos family, we all took pride in showing our perfectly clean teeth and cobs after eating. So just like our clients, we've always been huge fans of corn—fresh off the cob, canned, or frozen. The simple addition of the sweet, crisp kernels of corn can revolutionize any salad, jazzing it up, turning drab to fab. What's more, corn's complex carbohydrates provide long-lasting fuel for your brain and muscles, giving you energy and helping to fight off cravings for hours.

Most people don't realize that corn is a nutrient powerhouse. Corn is a starchy vegetable, so people think they should avoid it. This is a HUGE misconception. Corn isn't a source of empty calories; it is packed with nutrients and antioxidants. The reason that corn provides such chewing satisfaction is its high fiber content—both soluble (the kind that lowers cholesterol and blood sugar levels) and insoluble (the kind that prevents constipation). If you want to avoid the unsightly gut bulges from constipation and have energy to boot, corn is your ticket! The fiber in corn helps with blood sugar control and combines with its protein (corn has about 5 to 6 grams per cup) to even out the pace of digestion, thereby providing a steady supply of energy. When sugar enters the blood at a steady pace, you avoid sudden spikes and crashes in blood sugar. In addition to the fiber and protein in corn, its B-complex vitamins, including vitamins B_1, B_5, and folic acid, make it an excellent food for blood sugar control and very helpful for diabetics.

Don't think that's all that soluble fiber in corn can do for you; it may also have colon-cancer-fighting ability. This is partially due to the soluble fiber that can be metabolized by intestinal bacteria into short chain fatty acids (SCFAs). This process helps support populations of friendly bacteria in the gut, which promotes overall health. The SCFAs also provide a direct supply of energy to the cells that line the large intestine,

allowing the intestinal tract to decrease our susceptibility to a range of conditions including type 2 diabetes, obesity, inflammatory bowel disease, colon cancer, and autoimmune disorders such as rheumatoid arthritis.

We grew up loving the traditional white and yellow corn, but we didn't know that there are many other varieties including blue, purple, and red corn, which each provide different healthful antioxidants and phytonutrients. For example, yellow corn is loaded with carotenoids such as lutein and zeaxanthin (hello, healthy eyes!), beta-carotene (¡hola! healthy skin and eyes—and healthy pregnancy for moms-to-be!),

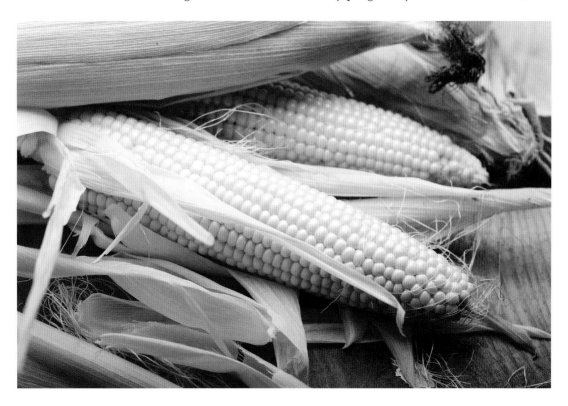

and beta-cryptoxanthin. Blue corn is rich in anthocyanins (welcome, flexible arteries and blood vessels). Corn's antioxidants as well as its fiber make it a heart-protective food that also lowers blood pressure and the risk for a wide variety of health problems and degenerative diseases. Eating corn is a good way to get the antioxidant nutrients, like vitamin C and manganese, that we've heard about since we were kids. Wanna join us in Edamame and Corn Salad for lunch, anyone?

Spotlight on Olives

Recipes with Olives: Edamame and Corn Salad, page 173; Fig and Olive Tapenade, page 135; Roasted Tomato Puttanesca, page 199

Around the corner from our homes in New York City is a store called Zabar's that's known for its specialty olives. Ask any foodie or tourist who comes to Manhattan's Upper West Side and they'll likely tell you that stopping in Zabar's for some olives and other delicacies is on their itinerary. Yes, people do travel for olives. Although more attention is often paid to the olive's delicious oil, these bite-size delicacies are one of the world's most widely enjoyed foods.

Although olives tend to be an acquired taste, after trying several different varieties in meals, it's easy to become an olive convert. This was certainly the case for us. It was a branzino with briny Greek Kalamata olives that converted us.

Olives add zest to your salad. If you crave a salty flavor, olives will quench your salt tooth, reducing the need for you to add any other source of sodium like bottled dressings to your salad.

Many olives start off green and turn black when fully ripe. However, some olives start off green or black and maintain their original color when fully ripe. Although some olives can be eaten right off the tree, most that you'd buy have been water cured, brine cured, or lye cured, which all affect the color and composition of the olive and reduce its natural bitterness. As dietitians, we're huge fans of all types of olives from both a flavor perspective and a health perspective. Interestingly, the different methods of olive preparation will provide a different concentration of antioxidant and anti-inflammatory nutrients. There are equal trade-offs that occur during olive ripening and olive curing. For instance, with advanced stages of ripening, the amounts of some phytonutrients like anthocyanins increase, yet those like oleuropein decrease. However, no matter what variety of olive you choose, you are always swallowing great flavor along with many delicious health benefits.

Do you shy away from olives because of their fat content? What you may not realize is that, aside from being packed with phytonutrients just like their oil, olives are a fabulous source of the heart-healthy monounsaturated fats. Olives

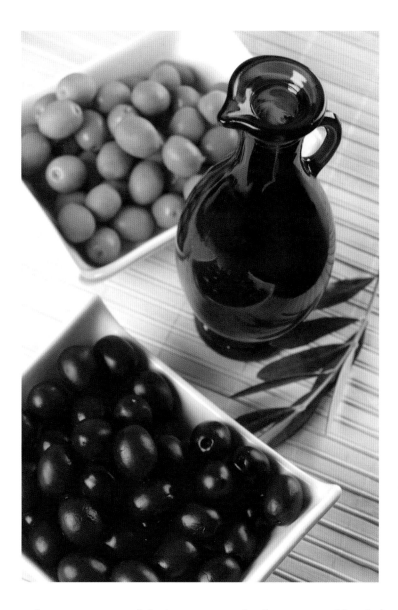

provide almost three-quarters of their fat as oleic acid, a monounsaturated fatty acid that actually lowers the risk of heart disease by decreasing blood pressure, blood cholesterol, and LDL cholesterol and improving the ratio of LDL to HDL. Think of olives helping your body to pump blood that delivers nutrients and oxygen throughout your body, benefiting your cardiovascular system—and helping you to get a speedy metabolism, gorgeous skin and hair and nails, and a well-functioning digestive system.

Oleic acid packs a double punch in our digestive tract by increasing our absorption of fat-soluble nutrients like carotenoids. This means that when you add olives to a salad, they act as a "nutrient booster," helping you to absorb a range of health-promoting fat-soluble nutrients like vitamins A (carotenoids), E, D, and K from the other veggies in the salad, like spinach, carrots, beets, and bell peppers. So olives work in tandem with other foods in your salad to keep you healthy, boost your immunity, make your skin smooth, and lift your mood. When you consider that olives also aid in fighting a wide range of diseases, including cancer, you begin to realize what gems they are. Olives also contain vitamin E, a powerful antioxidant that helps to "mop up" damaging free radicals in our body. The fat in the olives actually helps to enhance the absorption of the vitamin E found in the olives, further assisting in keeping you healthy, youthful, and disease-free.

Olives have an impressive phytonutrient content. It's rare to find high-fat foods that offer such a diverse range of antioxidant and anti-inflammatory nutrients. These antioxidant and anti-inflammatory phytonutrients are what cause olives to help almost all parts of the body. Olives' antioxidant and anti-inflammatory nutrients benefit the respiratory system, and powerful lungs mean you can exercise more efficiently and can more easily achieve a fit, healthy body. Olives' benefits even extend to the nervous system, the immune system, the digestive system (au revoir, low energy, constipation, and bloat), and the musculoskeletal system (¡hola! toned muscles and strong bones). New research shows that olives are great bone protectors. Yes, olives contribute to that sexy long and strong spine, the one that helps you to stand up straight and exude confidence! Thanks to hydroxytyrosol, an olive phytonutrient known to aid in cancer prevention, as well as oleuropein, the other key phytonutrient found in olives, olives are now recognized for helping to deposit calcium into the bone. Who knew? Roasted Tomato Puttanesca, anyone?

Do you suffer from allergies? Olives may help! Olive extracts have been shown to work as an antihistamine.

If you've been afraid to eat olives because you think of them as a high-fat food, keep in mind it's not artery-clogging saturated fat they are high in. They're high in monounsaturated fat, and it's time to recognize all of the health benefits that these fats have to offer! However, just like other high-fat plant foods that are high in monos (avocados, nuts, and seeds, for example), eat moderate portions so that you don't consume too many calories. Too many calories, no matter where they come from, cause weight gain.

CHAPTER 15

My Kid Won't Eat Veggies

Veggies Kids Will Love

The Problem: Your kids feed their veggies to the dog, hide them in their napkin, or simply refuse to eat them. A lack of healthful veggies leads to a lowered immunity and makes them more likely to catch a cold or the flu, as well as putting them at risk for other health issues.

Here's What You Need: Veggies that will put a lid on mealtime drama—ones that your kids will beg for, that are fun to eat (served with favorite dips, cut into fun shapes, or served on skewers) or that feel like comfort foods, but that are packed with the nutrients many kids' diets are low in (vitamins A, C, and E, calcium, fiber, magnesium, and potassium). Spaghetti squash, pumpkin, broccoli, cauliflower, carrots, and sweet potatoes are great sources of these nutrients.

Here's Why: The princes and princesses of "ick" and "yuck" typically fall far short on their vitamin and nutrient requirements because they eat the same bland, non-nutritious foods day in and day out. Pasta and boxed mashed potatoes are typical staples. When picky palates are offered nutrient-rich vegetables in ways that are yummy and fun to eat, they gobble them up, getting what they need to grow healthy and strong. Healthy versions of classics really boost nutrient intake. The most nutrient-rich foods of all are fresh vegetables and fruits, and kids need the nourishment they provide for optimal health as well as for growth and development.

Here's How to Get It: Always offer veggies to your kids at dinner. The secret is to try a variety of vegetables and experiment with different preparation methods. For example, you may find that your child doesn't like cooked carrots but likes raw carrots or simply has more fun eating baby carrots with a light dip. Or he or she may prefer fresh sautéed green beans to frozen green beans.

Realize that it may take 20 times for a child to become accepting of a new veggie, so don't give up. Your kids may turn up their noses at first, but eventually they will grow to accept a variety of vegetables if they are exposed enough times. Give a small, manageable portion (or even a bite) of a new vegetable. If your kid won't eat it, don't make a big deal out of it, but make sure you keep putting it on their plate so they can experiment with it. Kids are curious, and they will eventually give it a try.

Nutrient:	Why Your Kids Want It:	Why It Works:	Veggies to Get It:
Vitamin A	To be speedy and powerful on the playground; to be like their favorite princess or superhero with glowing skin and healthy eyes	Aids growth and development, tissue and bone repair, healthy skin and eyes, and immune responses	Yellow-to-orange vegetables like carrots, yams, and squash and green beans too
Vitamin C	To rule the kickball court with their strong muscles	Promotes healthy strong muscles, connective tissue, and skin	Tomatoes and green vegetables like broccoli and bell peppers
Vitamin E	To not get sick when friends sneeze on them or when they put unwashed hands in their mouth	Is vital for a strong immune system	Leafy greens and avocados
Calcium	To play sports and be kids, taking spills, without accidents resulting in broken bones; to grow at normal rates like their friends	Helps build strong bones	Broccoli and leafy green vegetables including turnip greens, spinach, and kale (to supplement dairy products)
Magnesium	To focus at school and get good grades	Is important to 300 bodily functions of muscles, nerves, heart, and more; boosts the immune system; strengthens bones; improves memory and learning ability	Dark green vegetables like broccoli and spinach; potatoes, avocados, and white, black, and navy beans
Fiber	To avoid the discomfort of constipation; to be free to play with their friends without being moody and edgy	Keeps them "regular"; also reduces risk of high cholesterol, heart disease, and type 2 diabetes later in life	Artichokes, peas, broccoli, carrots, sweet corn, brussels sprouts, potatoes with skin, spinach, avocados—all vegetables
Potassium	To stay energized so they can run, play, and have fun	Helps maintain proper fluid balance and hydration, wards off high blood pressure, and supports strong bones	Potatoes and sweet potatoes, leafy vegetables like spinach and Swiss chard

You need to eat your veggies too! And that should be easy—find the health, energy, or beauty remedy that turns you on and pick your veggie potion. Kids learn from you. If you don't make it a priority to eat a balanced diet yourself, they won't either. So eat healthy together as a family!

Spotlight on Broccoli

Recipes with Broccoli: Bangin' Broccoli East Meets West Style, page 209; Cauliflower and Broccoli Flapjacks, page 115; Cream of Whatever Soup, page 159; Hickory Broccoli Salad, page 175; Roasted Garlic Broccolini, page 232; Slam, Bam, Thank You Ma'am 5-Minute Broccoli or Cauliflower, page 235

We're not quite sure when our broccoli obsession began. We've both been hooked for as long as we can remember. However, Tammy's daughters are now being influenced by our obsession as well. Every night before dinner, they start their meal off with a veggie platter, and broccoli is always the first that her daughter Summer gobbles up.

One of the best things that you can do for your kids is getting them to eat broccoli. We call broccoli the gateway vegetable because once kids like and accept this green veggie, they are more likely to give others a bite, and their openness and willingness to try other veggies snowballs. Hallelujah!

It shouldn't be a shocker that broccoli is one of the most common and popular vegetables in America. Just watch a kid eat broccoli and you'll see why it's so easy for them to like. Their little fingers pinch off the small stems around the flower end, one by one like petals of a daisy, and then they pop the flower portion into their mouth. Add a dip or dressing for them to dunk the flower in, and you might as well start stocking up daily! If there's one veggie that provides most of the nutrients that vegetables can offer and that kids need for good health, it's broccoli. Plus, broccoli seems to have such a variety of benefits that witnessing your kids swallow it should make you feel like you are doing something incredible for them. Just don't overcook it; it will lose its nutrients, be mushy, and make quite a stink!

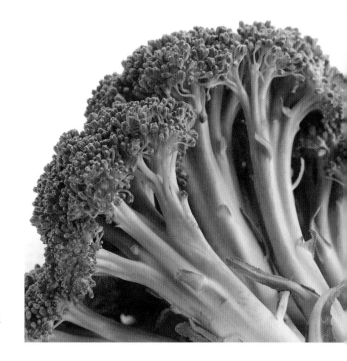

Based solely on its vitamin and mineral content, broccoli is a leader when it comes to what kids need. It's one of the best sources of vitamin C, which is something school-age children really need, especially when surrounded by so many germs. It's also one of the highest sources of vitamin A, which is needed for kids' normal growth and development, tissue and bone repair, and healthy skin, eyes, and immune responses. Broccoli contains a significant amount of calcium, which is necessary for strong, growing bones. Although it takes 4 cups of cooked broccoli or about five raw stalks to get the calcium provided by a cup of milk, cooked or raw it contributes to kids' calcium requirement. And broccoli's plentiful vitamin K also helps with the formation of a strong skeleton by "gluing" calcium to the bones. In addition, vitamin K helps blood to clot, so kids can form a scab after playground injuries. Plus, broccoli is a fantastic supplier of folate, fiber, potassium, and manganese. So the healthy growth and development of tissues, bones, muscles, eyes, and skin are just part of the allure of these stupendous stalks.

As a parent, it's a relief to know that you've got all of your bases covered. Broccoli will even help your little ones fight constipation. In fact, they'll get 1 gram of dietary fiber for every 10 calories—that's less than one-fifth of a cup! So for 50 calories (less than a cup of steamed broccoli) they'll get 5 grams of fiber. For a two- to three-year-old who may need only 14 grams of fiber a day, that broccoli will almost meet their daily needs. And it's almost half of the daily fiber requirement for kids and preteens! Broccoli's fiber also contains glucosinolates. These protect the health of the stomach lining by preventing bacterial overgrowth of *Helicobacter pylori* and by keeping the bacterium from clinging to our stomach wall.

Broccoli does it all, including fighting diseases like diabetes, depression, heart disease, stroke, and Alzheimer's, as well as helping to detox the body. It's never too early to start fighting heart disease or cancer, or to start activating the body's natural detox systems, and kids who eat their broccoli are off to a running start on all of these fronts. And when it comes to fighting cancer, broccoli is a superstar. Research has linked broccoli to a decrease in all types of cancer, especially showing the strongest decreased risk of prostate, colon, breast, bladder, and ovarian cancer.

Wonder how much fiber your kid needs each day? For a ballpark figure, take their age and add five. You'll get the number of grams of fiber your child should aim for every day.

Broccoli is packed with additional antioxidants other than vitamin C. It's these flavonoids, like kaempferol and quercitin, and the carotenoids lutein, zeaxanthin, and beta-carotene, as well as vitamin E and the minerals manganese and zinc, that make broccoli such a formidable free radical fighter.

Aim to start eating cruciferous veggies like broccoli as a family a minimum of two to three times a week, and make the serving size half a cup or more. Ideally, aim to eat them four to five times a week and increase the serving size to one or one-and-a-half cups or more. For kids, start slowly. Try small portions for children who typically don't get much fiber, and gradually increase their vegetable intake.

Steaming, boiling, or microwaving—what's the best way to retain broccoli's nutrients? Steaming. Use a low cooking temperature, steaming around 212°F (100°C), with a cooking time of five minutes at the most. Fill the bottom of a steamer pot with two inches of water. Steam broccoli stems for two minutes before adding the florets and leaves. Steam for five more minutes.

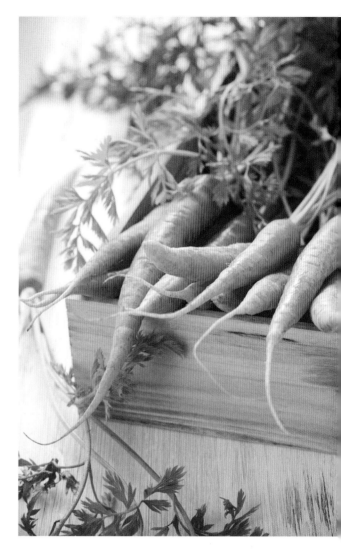

Spotlight on Carrots

Recipes with Carrots: Beet and Carrot Savory Pancakes, page 114; Carrot Zucchini Muffins, page 128; Honey Ginger Carrot Coins, page 223; Hot Diggity Chili!, page 195; Kung Pao Veggies, page 227; Quinoa with Mixed Vegetables, page 193; Split Pea and Barley Soup, page 166; Vegetable Broth, page 164; Vegetable Ribbons, page 239

At our house, family dinners always started with a green salad. Even before we could barely see above the table, we remember sitting down and immediately digging our little fingers through our salad to find carrot "coins." It was like finding treasure. As soon as we'd find them, we'd stuff one in our mouths and start crunching away while we'd hold another one up to our eyes, pretending we had carrot eyes, or pretending we were rich with all of our "money."

It's no wonder that we liked carrots so much; most kids do. They're crunchy, sweet, colorful, and ideal for dipping. So they do a lot of the work for us as parents. Instead of our having to try to force our kids to eat their veggies, carrots lure kids in. This is more important than most of us realize. When kids eat healthfully on their own, without a struggle, it takes the pressure off both them and their parents, and allows children to learn how to enjoy healthy foods. Any vegetable that makes our job as parents easier is a winner in our book. Plus, it turns out that carrots are excellent for kids (although all vegetables are great!).

Carrots are vitamin-A superheroes. In fact, they're one of the best sources of beta-carotene, which is converted to vitamin A in the body. A half cup of cooked carrots contains over 13,000 IUs of vitamin A. For children under 10, that's more than double their daily requirement! So a handful of baby carrots and your little boys and girls will be well on their way to being their favorite idol with beautiful skin and hair, and feeling like superheroes when they play tag with their friends. Because vitamin A is so crucial to growth and development, when your kids are chomping their carrots you can feel good knowing that those orange snacks are helping them to grow strong.

Thanks to their fiber content (3.6 grams in a cup of carrot strips), carrots will help to keep your little ones regular, eliminating grumpiness and temper tantrums due to discomfort. Crunching on carrots will help your kids get a very good dose of bone-building vitamin K, immunity-strengthening vitamin C, and potassium, great for keeping their hearts healthy and helping with muscle contraction.

All parents wants to do everything they can to keep their kids healthy. By giving your kids carrots, you are doing just that. In fact, new research shows that people who eat more than one-quarter cup of carrots a day have significantly lower risk of cardiovascular disease than those who eat less. Eat a serving of our Honey Ginger Carrot Coins or have your kids dip baby carrots in our Artichoke Hummus (page 126) and they'll easily get double! And new research shows that carrots are potent in helping to prevent the growth of colon cancer; when it comes to fighting cancer, carrots are stars.

Think that boiling your carrots destroys their nutrients? Not so! In fact, cooking carrots actually increases their beta-carotene and makes it more easily absorbed by the body.

CHAPTER 16

More Bang per Bite

Veggie Duos That Enhance Nutrient Absorption

These veggie combos can combat inflammation and free radical damage or simply enhance the absorption of nutrients. Each vegetable contains nutrients that are strong on their own but pack an even greater punch in tandem. This is especially important if you continuously fall short in meeting your recommended daily vegetable servings, or if, despite your best intentions, you don't always eat as nutritiously as you should.

The Problem: Like most people, you're not hitting your daily vegetable quota, and therefore you're not getting enough of the nutrients that you need to ensure your maximum health, beauty, and energy potential. You need to eat more veggies to increase your energy, combat wrinkles and the signs of aging, and help ward off disease. Pairing these foods together as power couples will ensure that the veggies on your plate are giving you the most antioxidant-rich, health-promoting bang for your bite.

Here's What You Need: Vegetables that contain phytonutrients that work synergistically with other plant foods to provide even greater health benefits than either one does on its own, not to mention that particularly please the palate when eaten together: tomatoes and avocados, red peppers and spinach, onions and rhubarb, to name just a few power couples.

Here's Why: Even though we may be biased when we say two doubles the fun, from a nutrient and flavor standpoint, one at a time is not the ideal way to get your vegetables. Antioxidant protection includes many nutrients and phytonutrients, and you need all of them for maximum effect. Additionally, the nutrients in some vegetables help you absorb nutrients in others, so eating them in combination can mean less inflammation and tissue damage or stronger bones and increased energy.

Here's How to Get It: Here are the combos that work and why:

Tomatoes and Avocados (lycopene and monounsaturated fat)
See Cold Cucumber and Avocado Soup, page 160; Guacamole Stuffed Tomato Poppers, page 140; Hole-in-One, page 116; and Ole! Mexican Cabbage with Black Beans and Avocados, page 179.

Tomatoes contain lycopene, a powerful antioxidant that helps prevent free radical damage, disease, and wrinkles. Diets high in lycopene have also been linked with lower risk of certain cancers. Cooked tomato products like tomato sauce, ketchup, tomato soup, and tomato paste are the best sources of lycopene, as the antioxidant concentration is significantly boosted and better absorbed by the body when cooked or processed.

Want to get even more lycopene bang per bite? Combine lycopene-rich foods like tomatoes with heart-healthy, mono-unsaturated-fat-rich avocados and you'll enhance the absorption of lycopene. A study at Ohio State University showed that people soak up over four times more lycopene when they eat it with avocado. One cup of fresh avocado (150 grams) added to a salad of romaine lettuce, spinach, and carrots increased absorption of carotenoids (lycopene is a carotenoid) by 200 to 400 percent.

> **Other good sources of lycopene: red carrots, papayas, watermelon, pink grapefruit, and guava.**

Bell Peppers and Spinach (vitamin C and iron)
See Dieter's Delight Chock Full of Veggies Soup, page 163, and Veggie Yard Dash Salad, page 183.

Feeling low on energy? You could be low in iron; the body needs iron to carry oxygen to your muscles and tissues for energy. The iron found in plants like chickpeas and dark leafy greens is nonheme iron (heme iron is found in meat and seafood). Nonheme iron isn't as easily absorbed by the body as heme iron, which is where vitamin C comes in. Foods high in vitamin C (bell peppers, broccoli, citrus fruits, strawberries) help increase the absorption of nonheme iron. So, to absorb the iron in spinach, eat it with bell peppers or broccoli. In fact, any time you have a veggie with iron in it (think spinach, beans, Swiss chard, even potatoes), combine it with a food rich in vitamin C (think tomatoes, onions, peppers, brussels sprouts, cauliflower) to enhance the absorption of the iron. So if you're prone to iron-deficiency anemia—many women are!—look for recipes in this book with the "power2" symbol and check to see if it's a duo rich in iron and vitamin C!

Note: Polyphenols, phytates, and calcium, components that naturally exist in tea, coffee, whole grains, legumes, and milk or dairy products, can decrease the amount of nonheme iron absorbed at a meal. Calcium can also decrease the amount of heme iron absorbed at a meal.

Leeks (or onions and garlic) and Greens (inulin and calcium)
Try our Herbed Pea Soup with Spinach, page 165, and Just Call Me Baby Bok Choy, page 228—a match made in veggie heaven.

Stronger bones are just a bite away. Inulin, a component of chicory-root plants, Jerusalem artichokes, onions, leeks, and garlic, helps improve calcium absorption. This means that some tasty combinations, like endive, the leaf of the inulin-rich chicory plant, and calcium-rich edamame, will help strengthen your bones with each bite. Other calcium-rich foods to try include bok choy, broccoli, and kelp.

Onions and Rhubarb (quercetin and catechin)

Try our Arugula Salad with Strawberry Rhubarb Vinaigrette, page 168.

When it comes to matters of the heart, think of tear-inducing onions and bright red rhubarb. The phytochemical quercetin found in onions, shallots, leeks, and scallions (also in apples and berries) and the catechins found in rhubarb (also in apples, green tea, and purple grapes) work together to help keep your heart safe. They prevent platelets from forming clots that can lead to a heart attack.

Antioxidants like Vitamin C and Vitamin E

Next time you eat our Easy Spinach Pomodoro (page 214), you can not only enjoy the pleasure on your palate but also take satisfaction in knowing that the vitamin E–rich spinach and the vitamin C–packed tomato sauce are teaming up to protect your heart. Vitamins C and E work in synergy to slow the oxidation of cholesterol. Remember, preventing the oxidation of cholesterol is critical, since cholesterol becomes dangerous only when it is oxidized. That's when cholesterol sticks to the arteries, gets inflamed, and causes the damage that results in heart disease, heart attack, and stroke.

Broccoli and Tomatoes

If you eat broccoli on its own, there's no doubt that you're doing something healthy for your body. Eat tomatoes on their own, and you're getting fiber and nutrients as well as powerful phytonutrients. But eat the broccoli and the tomatoes together, and now we're really talking. Research shows that prostate tumors grow much less in animals that are fed tomatoes and broccoli than in animals that eat diets containing broccoli alone or tomatoes alone.

(Perfect pairing quick tip: Simply add broccoli florets to chunky marinara sauce.)

Phytonutrients in a pill? If you skip your veggies, you may think you can make up for it by taking an antioxidant supplement. Not so. It's the whole vegetable (or fruit) that supports our health best, not supplements.

Spotlight on Avocados

Recipes with Avocados: Arugula Salad with Strawberry Rhubarb Vinaigrette, page 168; Cold Cucumber and Avocado Soup, page 160; Grapefruit, Avocado, and Kale Salad with Pepitas, page 174; Green Minted Cocoa Detox Smoothie, page 110; Guacamole Stuffed Tomato Poppers, page 140; Hole-in-One, page 116; Holy Fruity Guacamole!, page 144; Ole! Mexican Cabbage with Black Beans and Avocados, page 179; Sweet Potato Veggie Burgers, page 203

Avocados are known as a great addition to practically any meal because of their luscious, creamy texture and their ability to pair up well with almost all foods. So it shouldn't be any surprise that avocados appear on many wedding menus, including the salad served to Tammy's guests at her wedding. While your mouth enjoys the pleasing texture of an avocado, when it's paired with other vegetables, your entire body can also enjoy the health benefits of this tasty food. (Although avocados are technically fruits, we have categorized them here as a vegetable, since this is how they are usually considered from a culinary perspective.) If you've been fooled by the avocado's bad rap as a high-fat food, it's time to recognize all of the health benefits that these fats have to offer! But just like other high-fat plant foods (nuts and seeds, for example), eat moderate portions so that you don't consume too many calories. Too many calories, no matter where they come from, cause weight gain.

Avocados are rich in oleic acid. Not only does oleic acid lower the risk of heart disease, but it packs a double punch in our digestive tract by increasing our absorption of fat-soluble nutrients like carotenoids. This helps you absorb the impressive range of health-promoting carotenoids in the avocado itself, and it also means that avocados act as a "nutrient booster," increasing the absorption of fat-soluble nutrients provided by other foods. When they are paired with any other vegetable that contains fat-soluble nutrients like vitamins A (carotenoids), E, D, or K, they enhance your body's ability to absorb these important nutrients. When avocados are paired with lycopene-rich tomatoes, the carotenoid is more efficiently absorbed. Remember, carotenoids have antioxidant abilities and help boost the immune system, so combining them with avocado's oleic acid boosts your ability to reap their benefits. ¡Ole!

Avocados alone are still quite the catch. In fact, they immediately capture taste buds; the rich and creamy texture is such a delectable comfort food that even kids fall in love at first bite. Nutrient-loaded avocados are often one of a child's first foods because they are so pleasing on the palate.

Avocados are probably best known for their healthy monounsaturated fat. (Most people have never heard of oleic acid, so they wouldn't even realize that this is what makes up a lot of the monounsaturated fat content in avocados.) In

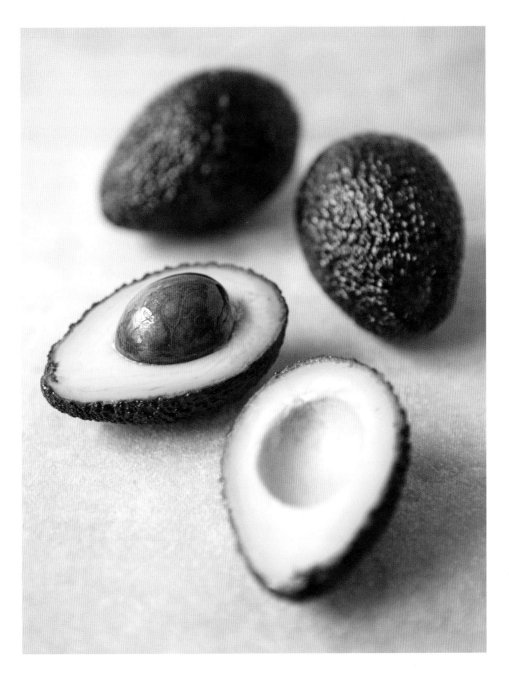

addition, a large percentage of the avocado's fat comes from phytosterols and polyhydroxylated fatty alcohols (PFAs), both of which are incredibly important in keeping inflammation under control. Find a way to kiss inflammation good-bye, and along with it goes most other health issues, like chronic diseases and aging skin. The phytosterols in avocados seem to be particularly helpful in fighting arthritis.

Another reason avocados can help combat inflammation and the unappealing health and beauty effects that follow? That would be the avocado's amazing carotenoid diversity. Despite the common belief that carotenoids are found only in bright orange or red vegetables like carrots or tomatoes, avocados, despite their dark green skin, contain an impressive range of carotenoids. And soon schoolkids will learn that the avocado is important for healthy vision, thanks to its carotenoids like beta-carotene, alpha-carotene, and especially the antioxidant lutein, which is concentrated in the macula of the eye. Research suggests that lutein helps maintain healthy eyesight as we get older. An ounce of avocado contains 81 micrograms of lutein; that is more than in an ounce of carrots.

Other special features of the avocado: Their alpha- and beta-carotene not only act as free radical scavengers, but they're also needed for proper growth and reproduction. Plus, avocados are packed with nearly 20 vitamins, minerals, and phytonutrients, many of which protect your heart, like vitamins E and C, folate, fiber, and potassium, as well as monounsaturated fat.

Peel the Skin, Keep the Nutrients

Want to ensure you get the most nutrients from your avocado? Use the nick-and-peel method. Since the greatest concentration of carotenoids in avocado is in the dark green flesh that is just beneath the skin, this method prevents you from slicing into that dark green portion any more than necessary. The first step in the nick-and-peel method is to cut into the avocado lengthwise, producing two long avocado halves that are still connected in the middle by the seed. Next, take hold of both halves and twist them in opposite directions until they naturally separate. Then remove the seed and cut each of the halves lengthwise so that you have long quartered sections of the avocado. Grip the edge of the skin on each quarter and peel it off, just as you would do with a banana skin. And voilà, you have a peeled avocado that contains most of that dark green outermost flesh, so rich in beneficial carotenoids!

Spotlight on Bell Peppers

Recipes with Bell Peppers: Asian Lettuce Wrap with Hoisin-Ginger Dipping Sauce, page 170; Colorful Crunch Salad with Honey Dijon Vinaigrette, page 169; Golden Gazpacho in Petite Cucumber Cradles, page 139; Roasted Red Pepper, Spinach, and Feta Portobello Burger, page 196; Veggie Frittata Bites, page 121

What's sweet and crunchy and our favorite snack-time veggie? Red bell peppers! We'd happily gobble up any bell pepper—green, yellow, orange, purple, black, or brown. We don't discriminate, and, yes, they come in all of those colors! We love that they are sweet and refreshing and that their crisp crunch satisfies that urge to chomp. Although the list of bell peppers' health attributes is long, when it comes to a match made in veggie heaven, their incredibly high vitamin C content is what beats out the competition. That's because you can boost the iron absorption in a vegetable when you eat it with a food that is high in vitamin C. This is huge. The iron that is found in vegetables is not easily absorbed, so you could consume an iron-rich vegetable like spinach and actually miss out on the veggie's high iron content. If you don't get enough iron, you'll feel tired and weak, as your muscles and tissues won't be able to get the oxygen they need. Not so when you add bell peppers; one cup provides a whopping 190 percent of the daily value for vitamin C, and a half- cup of raw red bell pepper contains about 50 percent more vitamin C than a medium-size orange. You can boost the iron absorption and actually reap the benefits of having more energy by simply adding this delectable vegetable to your spinach salad, stir-frying it with collards, or eating it with any iron-rich plant food like beans.

Recent research has shown that the vitamin C and carotenoid content as well as the total antioxidant capacity of bell

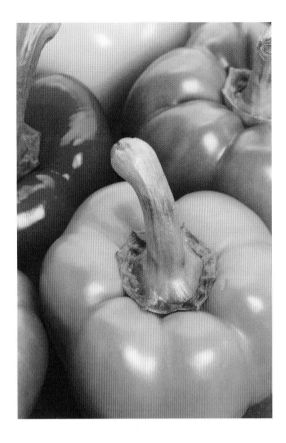

peppers tends to increase while the pepper is reaching its optimal ripeness. Bell peppers are also typically more flavorful when optimally ripe. Bell peppers can still ripen after they are picked. So how do you know if a pepper is at its peak for ripeness? Although it can be difficult to tell, a good rule of thumb is to judge by how vibrant in color it is, as well as its overall texture and feel. No matter what color, a ripe pepper will have deep, vivid color, feel heavy for its size, and be firm enough to give only slightly to pressure.

Not only do bell peppers make the perfect match with iron-rich plant foods, they are also an excellent source of antioxidant and anti-inflammatory phytonutrients, and contain more than 30 different members of the carotenoid nutrient family. This is impressive. Like vitamin C, carotenoids are powerful antioxidants, protecting the cells of your body from damage caused by free radicals. Carotenoids, and specifically beta-carotene, are also believed to enhance the function of the immune system and recently are getting a lot of attention as potential anticancer and antiaging compounds.

Bell Peppers' Key Nutrients

- Vitamin C

- Vitamin A

- Fiber

- Vitamin E

- Folate

- Potassium

- Vitamin K

- Molybdenum

- B vitamins

- Manganese

- Magnesium

- Lutein

Think it's best to chuck out the pulpy white inner cavity of the bell pepper? It's actually rich in flavonoids and can be eaten. We do!

Of all the cooking methods we've tried when cooking bell peppers, our favorite is simply a healthy "sauté." We think that it provides the greatest flavor and is also a method that allows for concentrated nutrient retention.

To "sauté" bell peppers, heat three tablespoons of water or low-sodium chicken or vegetable broth in a skillet. When bubbles begin to form, add sliced peppers, cover, and cook on medium heat for three minutes. After three minutes, add two tablespoons of water or broth and turn the heat to low. Cook uncovered while stirring for another four minutes.

Betcha didn't know that paprika is actually a dried and powdered form of bell pepper. Although you may only be familiar with red paprika, paprika can be made from any color bell pepper, and it will end up that same color once dried and ground into powder.

PART II

recipes

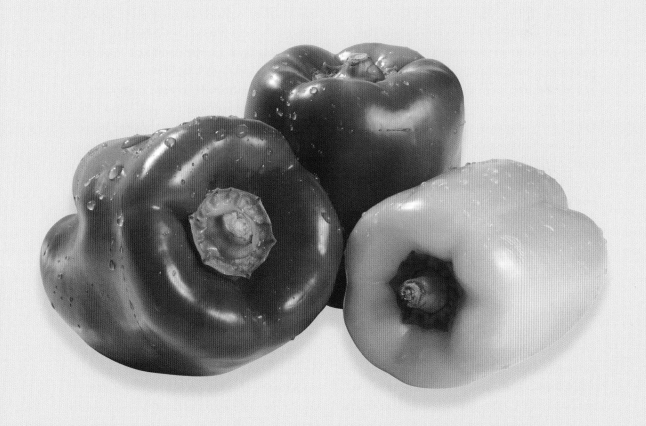

CHAPTER 17

The Nutrition Twins' Veggie Cure Recipes

Getting More Bang for Your Veggie Bite

Get the most flavor and health out of our recipes with these tips:

Salt: You'll notice that our recipes are very low to moderate in salt, and that in some recipes we note that you should salt to taste—and sometimes we say this is optional. Everyone has a different salt palate. The less salt you eat in your diet, the lower your preference for it, since your taste buds adjust to the amount they are given. Use less salt in your food, and your taste buds will quickly adapt and you'll need less salt in your food. You'll improve your health and your energy, and you'll look better too.

Salt increases inflammation in the body, so it doesn't just increase the risk for heart disease and high blood pressure, it also increases the risk of other chronic diseases, as well as speeding up the aging process and bloating you while increasing your cravings, making you hungrier and thirstier and your fat cells denser. Not good! That's why we wrote *The Secret to Skinny: How Salt Makes You Fat,* to help people to get lean and still enjoy their food. The recommendations are to get less than 2,300 milligrams of sodium daily (the amount you'd get in a teaspoon of salt) for about half the population

and less than 1,500 milligrams daily for most other people. The majority of people get too much—about two times the recommendation.

That being said, *just a tiny sprinkle of salt* can add a lot of flavor to a dish. The key is to add salt just before serving so that it hits your taste buds immediately, and to know how much you are adding so that you can keep it in check. If you are like us and your palate has a low salt threshold, then you may find that many of the recipes that note "salt to taste" don't need any salt added at all. If you prefer more salt, take heed and add the salt in a slow progression until it suits you, so that you can add as little as possible.

A word of encouragement: Taste preferences develop soon after birth, and they continue to progress depending on the foods we're exposed to. If you were frequently exposed to salty meals, it's likely that you acquired a taste for them. The good news is that our taste buds, like all other cells in the body, experience "turnover," which means they continuously die and are replaced. So if you go on a low-sodium diet for several weeks, your new taste buds will adjust and you'll prefer less salty food. In fact, it normally takes about 21 days for your taste buds to turn over, so if you use the recipes in this book for the next three weeks for each of your meals without adding extra salt, your taste buds will have adjusted! And you'll love that you'll have fewer cravings, feel less bloated, experience less under-eye puffiness—and your insides will thank you too!

Salad dressing: We have a couple of delicious dressing recipes in this book— our Herbed Vinaigrette (page 184) and our Honey Dijon Vinaigrette (page 169)—and we always keep them around the house so that we can toss them on our salads or other veggies, like our Slam, Bam, Thank You Ma'am 5-Minute Broccoli or Cauliflower (page 235). Most bottled dressings are high in sodium, fat, and calories; these dressings are not, yet they are so delicious. Both our dressings contain less than 29 calories and 66 milligrams of sodium for two tablespoons. Many salad dressings can be more than 100 calories and 200 to 400 milligrams of sodium for the same serving. So our dressings will help to keep you lean and bloat-free. If you don't make these vinaigrettes, we suggest that you always keep your favorite low-sodium, low-fat dressing available so that you can use it to flavor any of our veggies whenever you don't want to use the dressing that the recipe may call for.

Vegetable broth: You will notice that several of our recipes call for vegetable broth. Simply "sautéing" veggies in a broth can add an incredible amount of flavor without adding the fat and calories that oils add. The caveat is that just one cup of many store-bought broths can give you close to two-thirds of your daily sodium allotment. Just thinking about that makes us bloated! So we make our own Vegetable Broth (page 164) and keep it frozen in ice cube trays so that we can add it as we need it to "sauté" veggies when called for in recipes. You can do the same. If you don't want to prepare broths, there are two low-sodium brands of broth that taste best and that we recommend keeping on hand: Edward & Sons Low Sodium Veggie Bouillon and Rapunzel Vegan Vegetable Bouillon, No Salt Added.

Spray bottle: As registered dietitians we've witnessed that one of the healthiest foods has also caused some of the most unwanted pounds to accrue. Olive oil. Just a tablespoon of it (or of any oil) has 120 calories. That's almost one-tenth of the total calories many women should get in an entire day if they would like to shed a few pounds—and that's before even eating! It's easy to pour several tablespoons of oil into your salad. That's why we suggest putting your oil in a spray bottle. This will spritz the oil, dispersing it so that you can use a lot less. You still get the flavor and texture while sparing your waist, hips, and thighs.

Microplane: Similar to the way that the spray bottle prevents the fat and calories from accruing from healthy oils, a microplane not only helps with portion control of flavorful foods like Parmesan cheese and chocolate, but it also makes these delectable foods fun to eat. By turning heavy, rich foods into light ones—think shredded coconut or shaved Parmesan—the microplane helps you to get a lot of flavor for a few calories. One ounce of a cheese like Parmesan, grated on a microplane, looks like a large enough serving for four if grated on top of pasta! If you don't have a microplane, you could find a good one online for about $12 at us.microplane.com, or you can use a zester.

Onions, garlic, shallots, leeks: Our recipes contain notes suggesting that after cutting vegetables in the allium family like onions, garlic, shallots, and leeks, you let them sit for at least five minutes before cooking or eating them to help enhance their health-promoting benefits. Here's why: The chopping or dicing ruptures the cells of the onions or other allium veggies and releases an enzyme, alliinase, that causes the formation of the cancer-fighting phytonutrient allicin. Since cooking can inactivate alliinase, the enzyme that starts it all, letting allium veggies stand for five to ten minutes after chopping or crushing will give you the health-promoting, cancer-fighting benefits you want.

Frozen vegetables: Frozen vegetables are just as healthy as fresh ones. In fact, in some instances, frozen are even healthier. Frozen vegetables are picked and frozen immediately, nutrients intact. Fresh vegetables may lose nutrients during shipping and storage, or when on the store shelves, when vegetables are exposed to light, heat, and air. You'll notice that several of our recipes call for frozen vegetables (although we give an option to use fresh vegetables as well). This not only ensures retention of nutrients, but it also helps to make meals quick and easy to prepare. You can keep frozen vegetables in your freezer for months—nearly up to a year!—so you never have to worry about not having vegetables if your fresh ones go bad.

Legend

These symbols appear throughout the recipe section to denote specific health benefits.

CODE:

heart | **fights heart disease**

can | **fights cancer**

bones | **strengthens bones**

kid | **kid-friendly**

skin | **enhances skin's beauty and helps prevent damage that ages skin**

slim | **helps make you lean and svelte**

detox | **cleanses and detoxes the body**

preg | **provides vital nutrients for pregnancy**

bloat | **fights bloat**

stress | **fights stress and the damage it creates**

full | **very satisfying meal**

mood | **enhances mood and well-being**

power2 | **enhances nutrient absorption and benefit of paired foods**

time | **fast, easy to prepare**

energy | **provides a power boost of sustained energy**

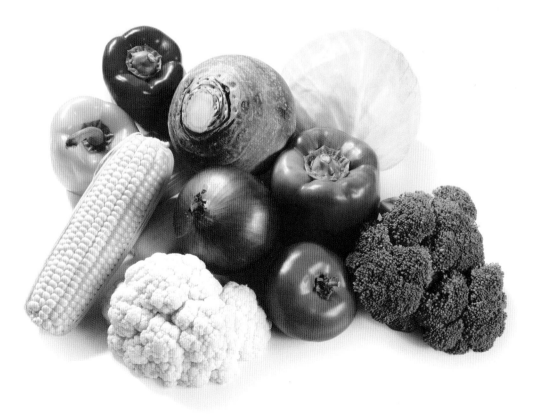

Berry Yogurt Detox Smoothie

heart | can | preg | bones | slim | bloat | skin | full | stress | mood

This sweet smoothie is light and makes a great energy-boosting breakfast or a refreshing snack. The berries and spinach pack an extra antioxidant punch, while the protein in the yogurt will keep you satisfied. If you've had a heavy meal last night and are paying the price with bloat, this liquid elixir will help to quickly rid the bloat and get you back on the lean and svelte track.

Variation: If you don't want to use milk and yogurt, you can replace them with roughly 130 calories of a high-protein alternative. This is generally 1⅓ scoops of whey protein powder. Then add 1 cup of ice and half a banana. Or if you're vegan you could use 5 tablespoons of hemp protein powder and 1 cup of ice and half a banana to replace the milk and yogurt. Please note that this will slightly change the viscosity and the flavor.

Serves 2 (8 ounces per serving)

½ cup skim milk

½ cup flavored, fat-free yogurt (we like fruit flavors, especially berries)

1 teaspoon honey

½ cup raw baby spinach, packed

½ teaspoon ground flaxseed (optional)

¼ teaspoon ground cinnamon

1 cup frozen strawberries, unsweetened

½ cup frozen blueberries, unsweetened

Combine all ingredients in a blender and puree until smooth.

Tip: We've found it's best to layer smoothie ingredients into the blender jar in the following order: liquid, spinach, spices, then frozen ingredients on top. This allows the blender to make a slurry with the liquids, which draws the frozen fruit down to the blades while keeping the blender from getting hung up on the frozen ingredients.

Variation: For an extra boost add ¼ cup walnuts. For best results soak the nuts in water for 15 minutes, drain, then add to the blender with the rest of the ingredients to process.

> Another reason this smoothie will give you a perk? It's got a dash of honey, a natural energizer that has long been used by athletes as a quick pick-me-up because of its carbohydrate count.

Per serving (not including optional flaxseed or walnuts): calories 150, total fat 1g, saturated fat 0g, cholesterol 2mg, sodium 76mg, carbohydrates 33g, dietary fiber 4g, sugars 26g, protein 6g
Percent Daily Value: vitamin A 16%, vitamin C 83%, iron 7%, calcium 20%

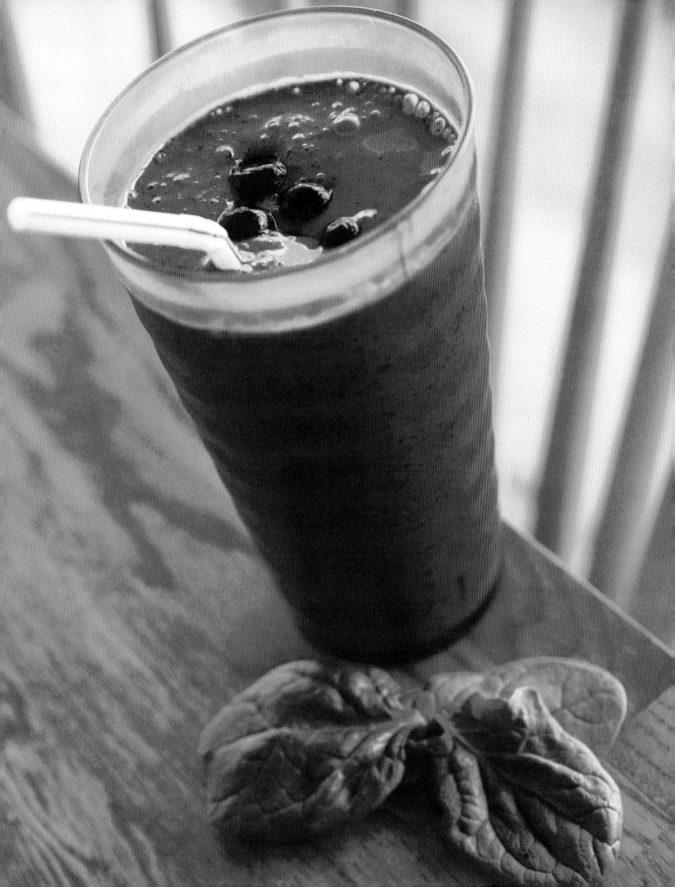

Fruity Green Smoothie

heart | can | preg | bones | slim | bloat | skin | full | stress | mood

We love that this sweet and refreshing thirst quencher is actually a bloat-be-gone drink packed with fiber and nutrients. Thanks to its high potassium and water content, this is is a great choice to flush out swelling sodium. Its fiber helps to keep your digestive tract free and clear. This makes a great, light afternoon snack after a high-salt lunch.

Serves 2 (10 ounces per serving)

1 cup liquid: either water, chilled unsweetened green tea, or coconut water

¾ cup raw baby spinach, packed

½ cup peeled and cubed cucumber

¼ lime, peel and pith removed

4 mint leaves (optional)

½ teaspoon ground flaxseed (optional)

⅛ teaspoon ground cardamom

Pinch of freshly ground black pepper

1 frozen banana, sliced

⅓ cup frozen pineapple

⅓ cup frozen mango

Combine all ingredients in a blender and puree until very smooth.

Tip: We've found it's best to layer smoothie ingredients into the blender jar in the following order: liquid, vegetables, spices, then frozen ingredients on top. This allows the blender to make a slurry with the liquids, which then draws the frozen fruit down to the blades while keeping the blender from getting hung up on the frozen ingredients.

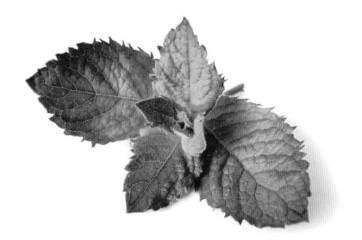

Per serving (prepared with coconut water, no flax): calories 129, total fat 1g, saturated fat 0g, cholesterol 0mg, sodium 138mg, carbohydrates 32g, dietary fiber 5g, sugars 19g, protein 3g
Percent Daily Value: vitamin A 28%, vitamin C 47%, iron 7%, calcium 6%

Greenana Apple Pear Smoothie

can | slim | bloat | stress | time | detox

This frothy drink provides a whopping antioxidant boost to help repair damaged cells. Using a slightly riper banana will allow its starch to become sweeter, and of course the sweeter your fruit, the sweeter the smoothie. If you are in need of a detox following a rough night, this smoothie is a great way to start your day with purifying kale. Enjoy it for a snack or pair it up with a hard-boiled egg or a nonfat yogurt for a healthy breakfast. It can be made in under five minutes!

Serves 4 (8 ounces per serving)

1. Place all ingredients in a large blender.

2. Blend until color is completely uniform and there are no more pieces.

1 banana

1 pear, chopped

1 apple, chopped

2 cups chopped kale, stems removed

1 cup chopped lettuce

1 tablespoon lemon juice

1 stalk celery, chopped

2 springs cilantro (optional)

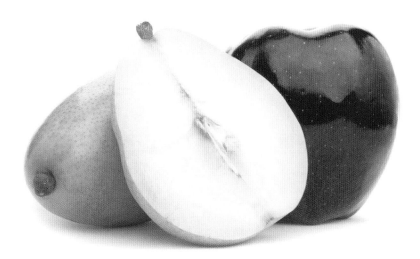

Per serving: calories 93, total fat 0g, saturated fat 0g, cholesterol 0mg, sodium 27mg, carbohydrates 23g, dietary fiber 4g, sugars 13g, protein 2g
Percent Daily Value: vitamin A 123%, vitamin C 84%, calcium 6%, iron 5%

Green Minted Cocoa Detox Smoothie

heart | can | preg | bones | slim | bloat | skin | stress | mood

This smoothie is one of our faves: One serving provides a perfect protein and fiber combo that makes an ideal low-calorie snack or breakfast. And if you really want to feel satisfied, you can have two servings for fewer than 250 calories—a wonderful, slimming, antioxidant- and protein-filled breakfast. The flavor reminds us of an Andes mint, which we are wild for. It's an invigorating and refreshing way to start the day. This smoothie is ideal for helping you to keep muscle tone when you are slimming down.

Variation: If you don't want to use Greek yogurt, you can replace it with roughly 130 calories of a high-protein alternative. This is generally 1⅓ scoops of whey protein powder. Then add 1 cup of ice. Or if you're vegan, you could use 5 tablespoons of hemp protein powder and 1 cup of ice to replace 1 cup of Greek yogurt. Please note that this will slightly change the viscosity and the flavor.

Serves 4 (8 ounces per serving)

¾ cup chopped ripe banana (1 medium banana)

¼ cup chopped green apple (½ medium apple)

1 teaspoon cocoa powder

1 cup raw baby spinach, packed

1 teaspoon flaxseed

½ cup chopped avocado (½ medium avocado)

1 cup unsweetened almond milk

1 cup nonfat Greek yogurt

2 tablespoons chopped fresh mint (about 6 leaves)

1 tablespoon fresh-squeezed lemon juice (juice from ½ lemon)

Chop the larger ingredients into smaller pieces to facilitate the blending process. Combine all of the ingredients in a blender and puree until smooth.

Note: If you don't like mint, you can replace the mint with basil. Although we personally prefer the mint, the basil adds a bright, fresh taste to complement the chocolate.

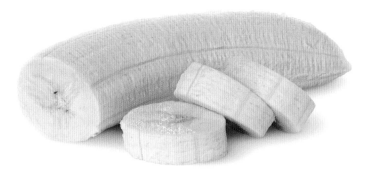

Per serving: calories 123, total fat 4g, saturated fat 0g, cholesterol 4mg, sodium 81mg, carbohydrates 16g, dietary fiber 4g, sugars 9g, protein 8g
Percent Daily Value: vitamin A 32%, vitamin C 20%, calcium 15%, iron 5%

Minted Mango Melon Detox Smoothie

can | slim | bloat | skin | heart | can | preg | bones | stress | mood

If you're looking for an easy-to-prepare and scrumptious meal to aid in your weight loss efforts, look no further. With less than 120 calories, this is the ideal slimming breakfast or satisfying snack. It provides a winning combo of protein and fiber to keep you satisfied and prevent you from over-eating at your next meal. The flavor is reminiscent of a creamsicle accented with fresh mint. One serving provides more than a day and a half of immune-boosting vitamin C and 130 percent of the daily value for vitamin A. Depending on your appetite, you may want to have two servings of this to make your entire breakfast. Go for it since it's so low in calories!

Variation: If you don't want to use Greek yogurt, you can replace it with roughly 130 calories of a high-protein alternative. This is generally 1⅓ scoops of whey protein powder. Then add 1 cup of ice. Or if you're vegan, you could use 5 tablespoons of hemp protein powder and 1 cup of ice to replace 1 cup of Greek yogurt. Please note that this will slightly change the viscosity and the flavor.

Serves 4 (12 ounces per serving)

Chop the larger ingredients into smaller pieces to facilitate the blending process. Combine all the ingredients in a blender and puree until smooth.

Note: If you don't care for mint, you can replace it with fresh basil, which will provide a different but also yummy flavor.

2 cups chopped cantaloupe

1 cup chopped cucumber

½ cup peeled and chopped kiwi (about 2 kiwi)

¼ cup fresh spinach, packed

½ cup mango, frozen pieces

¼ cup chopped mint leaves, (not packed)

1 tablespoon fresh-squeezed lemon juice

1 pinch of freshly ground black pepper

1 cup nonfat Greek yogurt

1 cup ice

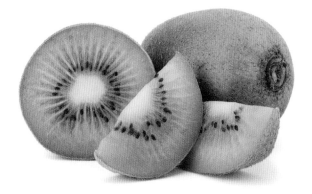

Per serving: calories 118, total fat 1g, saturated fat 0g, cholesterol 4mg, sodium 67mg, carbohydrates 22g, dietary fiber 4g, sugars 16g, protein 9g
Percent Daily Value: vitamin A 130%, vitamin C 152%, calcium 12%, iron 8%

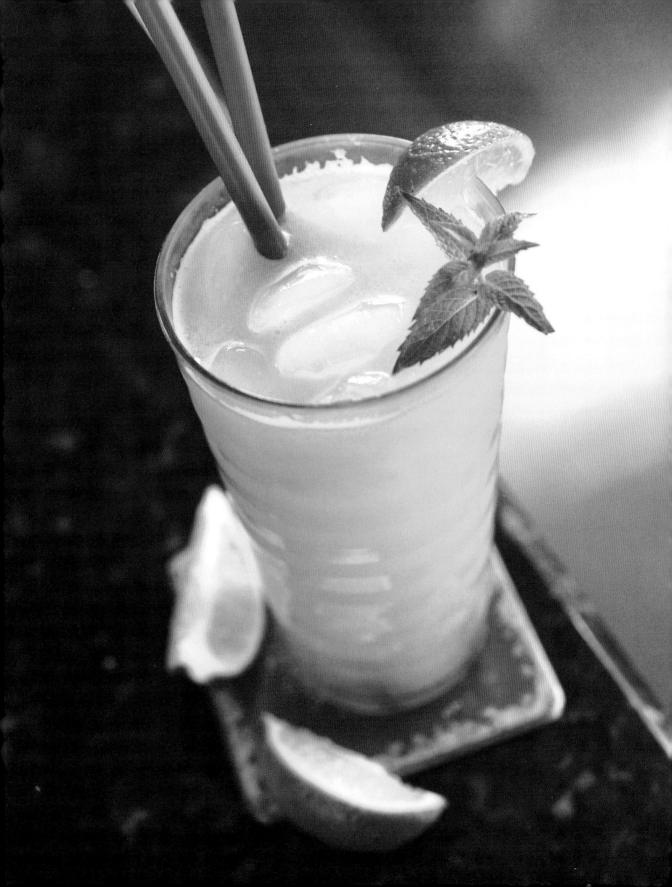

Sparkling Cucumber Detox and Refresher

can | slim | bloat | skin

When we wake up in the morning, the first thing we always do is hydrate with a big glass of water. On days when we feel like we need something to give us an extra lift, this refresher does the trick. We love a little bubbly boost, and for virtually zero calories per serving, we like that this starts our morning off by refreshing us. Drink this and you'll feel better if you've had too much salt the night before, as it helps fight bloat and under-eye puffiness. It also gives skin a bright hue.

Serves 4 (8 ounces per serving)

FOR JUICE:

1. Blend the chopped cucumbers in a food processor for 2 to 3 minutes, then pour the mash into a strainer placed over a bowl. Use a spatula to press the liquid from the pulp; this also makes the drink less frothy. For an even less pulpy liquid, use cheesecloth or coffee filters over your strainer.

2. Refrigerate.

FOR 1 SERVING OF SPARKLING CUCUMBER DETOX AND REFRESHER:

1. Fill a 12-ounce glass halfway with ice and then add 4 ounces of cucumber juice.

2. Add lime juice.

3. Top with 4 ounces of seltzer, or more if desired.

4. Add a wedge of lime and a mint sprig.

4 medium cucumbers, peeled and chopped (makes about 2 cups [16 ounces] of fresh cucumber juice)

Juice of ½ lime (about 1 tablespoon)

4 ounces lime seltzer (we use Polar Lime or Cranberry-Lime for an extra fruity twist)

Lime wedge and mint sprig (for garnish)

We like to keep the cucumber "broth" in the refrigerator, ready to go at all times.

Per serving: calories 8, total fat 0g, saturated fat 0g, cholesterol 0mg, sodium 2mg, carbohydrates 2g, dietary fiber 0g, sugars 0g, protein 0g
Percent Daily Value: vitamin A 4%, vitamin C 16%, calcium 4%, iron 4%

Beet and Carrot Savory Pancakes

heart | can | kid | bloat | skin | full | stress | mood | detox | bones | slim

Beets and carrots and apples, oh my! This recipe had us even before we knew these would be pancakes. This is the perfect way to start your day with a "cleansing" breakfast, packed with fiber for healthy digestion, beets for purification, and carrots to boost your immune system. Count us in!

Serves 4 (two 4-inch pancakes per serving)

1 clove garlic, minced

1 cup whole wheat flour

1 egg

1 teaspoon baking powder

1 cup nonfat Greek yogurt

½ cup grated beets

½ cup grated carrots

¾ cup grated Granny Smith apple

2 tablespoons chopped scallions

1 teaspoon Dijon mustard

¼ teaspoon freshly ground pepper

½ tablespoon chopped fresh rosemary

1 tablespoon grated fresh ginger

1 tablespoon fresh lemon juice

2–3 teaspoons canola oil

1 cup applesauce, for serving

1. Preheat the oven to 200°F.

2. Mince the garlic and allow it to sit for at least 5 minutes before cooking.

3. In a medium bowl, mix the flour, egg, baking powder, and the yogurt until a smooth, thin batter forms. Stir in the beets, carrots, apple, scallions, mustard, pepper, rosemary, ginger, and lemon juice. The batter will be thick and chunky.

4. Add 1 teaspoon of oil to a large nonstick pan over medium heat. When the pan is hot, drop in ⅓ cup batter, flattening it out into a 4-inch pancake. Cook for 2 to 3 minutes or until the top of the pancake looks slightly bubbly and dry. Turn and cook for another 2 to 3 minutes on the other side. Use the remaining teaspoon(s) of oil as necessary to cook the remaining pancakes.

5. Keep pancakes warm in the 200°F oven until all are cooked. Serve with a dollop of applesauce.

Per serving with ¼ cup applesauce topping each: calories 228, total fat 3g, saturated fat 0g, cholesterol 1mg, sodium 207mg, carbohydrates 45g, dietary fiber 6g, sugars 18g, protein 9g
Percent Daily Value: vitamin A 47%, vitamin C 9%, iron 10%, calcium 21%

Cauliflower and Broccoli Flapjacks

heart | preg | can | kid | slim | bloat | stress | mood | detox | bones | skin

These are one of our all-time favorites because they are so simple to make and so delicious to taste. They work for any meal, and they're one of the easiest ways to whip up vegetables that everyone will like. Starting with frozen veggies means you don't have to worry about fresh ones going bad. Plus, they are low in calories and packed with cancer-fighting nutrients. You can freeze them and then pop them in the microwave for a fast meal.

Serves 4 (two 3-inch flapjacks per serving)

1. Beat eggs together with flour until smooth. Add salt, minced onion, and pepper; cayenne is optional. Defrost broccoli and cauliflower and finely chop them. (If you need to hide vegetables for picky eaters, use a blender to finely chop them.) Add to batter. Mix well.

2. Heat a large skillet on medium-high and coat pan with canola oil spray. Using a ¼-cup measuring cup, and making sure to get enough egg and vegetables in each scoop, pour batter onto hot skillet and cook until bottom sides are golden brown, approximately 2 minutes. Then flip over and cook other side for 1 minute more. Re-spray pan before each set of pancakes.

3. Enjoy with some nonfat Greek yogurt or tzatziki sauce!

Tip: These savory pancakes are like a blank canvas that can go well with anything. You can serve them with yogurt, tzatziki sauce, salsa, or our Creamy Spinach Dip (page 134), although we like them as is, on their own.

2 eggs

2 tablespoons whole wheat flour

¼ teaspoon salt

2 tablespoons minced onion

½ teaspoon pepper

¼ teaspoon cayenne pepper (optional)

3 cups frozen mixed cauliflower and broccoli

Canola oil spray

Salt to taste (optional)

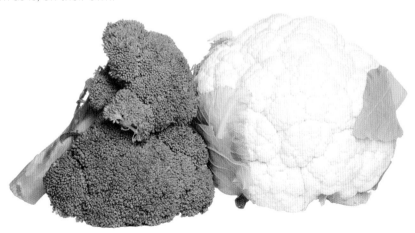

Per serving: calories 46, total fat 2g, saturated fat 1g, cholesterol 59mg, sodium 105mg, carbohydrates 4g, dietary fiber 2g, sugars 1g, protein 3g
Percent Daily Value: vitamin A 8%, vitamin C 48%, calcium 3%, iron 4%

Hole-in-One

heart | power2 | can | preg | kid | skin | bones | bloat | stress | mood

This is the perfect breakfast if you are tired of the same old thing and want something new that's scrumptious and satisfying. It's an all-time favorite for most who try it, and you get the good-for-you fats from the avocado and the lycopene from the tomatoes that will help to keep your heart and your skin healthy.

Serves 2

1 firm Hass avocado

1 egg or egg white

2 teaspoons finely chopped tomatoes

Salt to taste

1. Preheat oven to 425°F.

2. Split the avocado lengthwise and remove the pit with a spoon or knife. Cut a small section off the back of each avocado half so it lies upright. Place both halves on a baking sheet.

3. Crack the egg into a bowl, beat lightly, and split evenly between the two halves of avocado.

4. Top with tomatoes, put in oven, and bake for 25 minutes or until egg is done to your preference. Enjoy your breakfast with a slice of toast!

Bonus: This takes just minutes to throw together; the oven does the work for you. After 25 minutes you come back to a delicious meal.

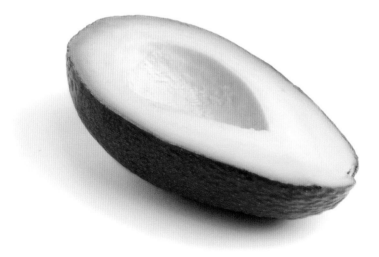

Per serving (using 1 extra-large egg, no salt): calories 156, total fat 13g, saturated fat 2g, cholesterol 118mg, sodium 45mg, carbohydrates 7g, dietary fiber 5g, sugars 1g, protein 5g
Percent Daily Value: vitamin A 7%, vitamin C 12%, calcium 2%, iron 5%

Pumpkin Pancakes

can | kid | skin | energy | full

Who doesn't love pancakes?! And this fabulous twist on the traditional pancake will fill you with just the right combination of carbohydrate, protein, and fiber to start your day with a burst of energy. The pumpkin gives a wonderfully fluffy texture to the pancake while supplying fiber, and the yogurt and cottage cheese add a boost of protein that keeps you feeling satisfied for hours without weighing you down.

Serves 5 (two 3⅓-inch pancakes per serving)

1. Beat eggs in a bowl and whisk in pumpkin, yogurt, and cottage cheese.

2. In another bowl mix together dry ingredients: flour and baking soda.

3. Add dry ingredients to wet ingredients and mix until well blended. Add applesauce for a moister pancake, or leave out if you prefer a more bread-like texture.

4. Spray griddle with canola oil.

5. Using a ¼-cup measuring cup, pour batter onto a hot griddle over medium heat. Spread in a circular motion with backside of spoon.

6. After approximately 3 minutes, when edges are slightly brown, flip pancakes to cook other side.

7. Top with applesauce (if desired).

2 eggs

½ cup canned pumpkin pie filling

½ cup nonfat Greek yogurt

⅓ cup cottage cheese (1%, no salt added)

¾ cup whole wheat flour

½ teaspoon baking soda

½ cup unsweetened applesauce (optional, preferable if you like a moister pancake)

Canola oil spray

½ cup unsweetened applesauce, for topping (optional)

Per serving (without any topping): calories 148, total fat 2g, saturated fat 0g, cholesterol 76mg, sodium 226mg, carbohydrates 26g, dietary fiber 4g, sugars 4g, protein 8g
Percent Daily Value: vitamin A 46%, vitamin C 10%, calcium 8%, iron 8%

Pumpkin 'n' Apple-y Yogurt Parfait

can | kid | skin | energy | full | time

We're pumpkin obsessed—it's hard not to be, as you know if you've tried our pumpkin pancakes, pumpkin quiche, or pumpkin muffins. Canned pumpkin with no salt added is one of the easiest ways to get a nutrient-packed veggie that adds a sweet creaminess to any meal. One-half cup has 40 calories and 350 percent of your daily vitamin A requirement (hello glowing, rejuvenated skin!). This pumpkin parfait is the perfect way to fuel your day with fiber and protein for long-lasting energy and is a great, satisfying way to start your morning.

Serves 2 (1 parfait each)

2 small Fuji apples, cored and sliced ¼–½ inch thick

2¼ teaspoons pumpkin pie spice mix (or ¼ teaspoon cloves, 1 teaspoon nutmeg, 1 teaspoon cinnamon), divided

2 teaspoons sugar

½ cup canned pumpkin without added salt

12 ounces nonfat vanilla yogurt (see note)

¼ cup cooked quinoa (optional)

1. Place sliced apple in a microwave-safe bowl and mix well with 2 teaspoons pumpkin pie spice mix. Microwave on high for 3½ minutes. Apples should be soft and juicy, as if you had baked them. Depending on your microwave, you may need to microwave for another minute or minute and a half.

2. While apple is cooking, in a medium bowl add sugar and remaining pumpkin pie spice to pumpkin and stir. When thoroughly combined, fold in the yogurt until evenly mixed throughout.

3. In each of two tall glasses, place 3 ounces of the yogurt-pumpkin mixture.

4. When apple finishes cooking, remove from microwave while still hot and place one-quarter on top of each pumpkin mixture in the glasses. Repeat by layering yogurt-pumpkin mixture with apples. Top with quinoa if you'd like.

Note: To keep sugar in check, look for yogurt with no more than 120 calories per 6-ounce serving.

Time-saver: Only got a minute to get out the door? Get a delish version of this nutrient-packed veggie breakfast by simply mixing ⅓ cup canned pumpkin with 1 teaspoon brown sugar and stirring in vanilla yogurt. Sprinkle with a dash of pumpkin pie spice. You can eat an apple on the side!

Per serving (without quinoa): calories 204, total fat 1g, saturated fat 0g, cholesterol 3mg, sodium 135mg, carbohydrates 41g, dietary fiber 5g, sugars 33g, protein 11g
Percent Daily Value: vitamin A 193%, vitamin C 18%, iron 7%, calcium 36%

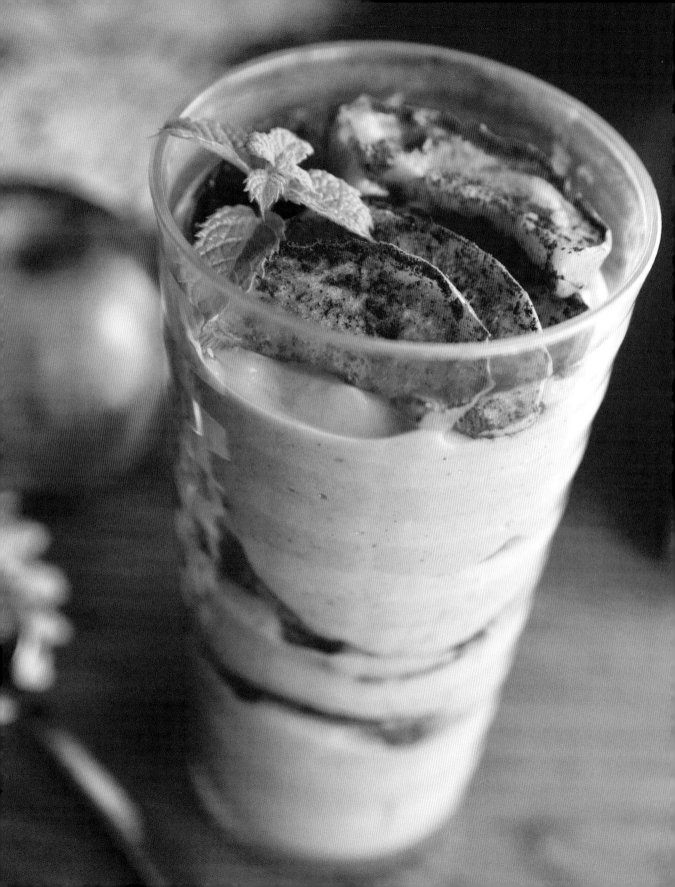

Sweet and Savory Pumpkin Quiche

heart | can | preg | bones | slim | skin | full | stress | mood | kid | energy

This delicious dish is the perfect mix of sweet and savory. You'll want it any time of day—it makes a great breakfast, lunch, or snack. Enjoy it hot and cold! We sure do!

Serves 8

Cooking spray

⅓ cup chopped sweet onion

1 cup chopped mushrooms

2 cups chopped spinach leaves

4 wedges Laughing Cow Light Creamy Swiss cheese

1 (15-ounce) can or 1¾ cups pureed pumpkin

1¼ cups fat-free liquid egg substitute

½ teaspoon nutmeg

½ teaspoon cinnamon

2 tablespoons brown sugar

Pinch of salt (optional)

1. Preheat oven to 350°F and grease a 9 x 9-inch casserole dish lightly with cooking spray.

2. Sauté onions in a lightly sprayed pan for 3 minutes until softened and lightly brown. Set aside in a small bowl.

3. In the same pan and on medium heat, sauté mushrooms for 4 minutes. Add spinach and sauté until spinach is wilted, another 2 minutes. With your spatula, break up Laughing Cow cheese and turn into mixture until it is completely melted.

4. In a separate bowl, place pumpkin and egg substitute and mix well with a whisk. Add onions and cheese-spinach mixture. Mix well and then add nutmeg, cinnamon, and brown sugar (and salt, if using).

5. Pour into casserole dish and even out with spatula. Bake for 1 hour in oven or until knife inserted in the center comes out clean. Cool before cutting, and serve as a side or as a light lunch.

Per serving (no salt added): calories 90, total fat 1g, saturated fat 0.5g, cholesterol 2mg, sodium 185mg, carbohydrates 10.5g, dietary fiber 2g, sugars 6.5g, protein 7g
Percent Daily Value: vitamin A 181%, vitamin C 8%, calcium 10%, iron 11%

Veggie Frittata Bites

bloat | skin | heart | bones | preg | can | kid | slim | stress | mood

These adorable bites are so easy to make ahead, freeze, and reheat! Grab one or two on your way out the door for a quickie breakfast with a piece of fruit, or have one for a snack. They're a delicious way to get your veggies, plus a fantastic filling protein that will keep you feeling satiated throughout the morning. And if you're looking to lose a few pounds, you'll love that you can fill up on these with few calories, thanks to all of the veggies combined with protein.

Yields 10 muffin-size servings

1. Preheat oven to 350°F.

2. Beat eggs, milk, pepper, and salt (if using) in medium bowl until blended. Add cheese, zucchini, tomato, mushrooms, bell pepper, and onion; mix well.

3. Using a ½-cup measuring cup, scoop and pour evenly into 10 lightly sprayed muffin cups. Bake until just set, 25 minutes. Cool on rack 5 minutes. Remove from cups by loosening sides with a knife, and serve warm.

6 eggs

½ cup skim or 1% milk

⅛ teaspoon freshly ground pepper

1 cup (4 ounces) low-fat or fat-free shredded cheddar cheese

½ cup chopped zucchini

½ cup chopped tomatoes

½ cup chopped mushrooms

½ cup chopped green bell pepper

2 tablespoons chopped red onion

Pinch of salt (optional)

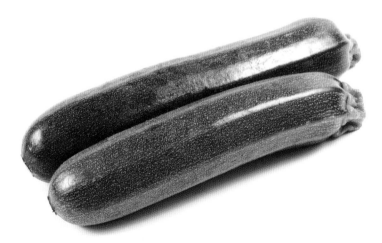

Per serving (with fat-free cheese and skim milk, no salt added): calories 70, total fat 3g, saturated fat 1g, cholesterol 143mg, sodium 220mg, carbohydrates 3g, dietary fiber 0g, sugars 2g, protein 7g
Percent Daily Value: vitamin A 9%, vitamin C 14%, iron 4%, calcium 14%

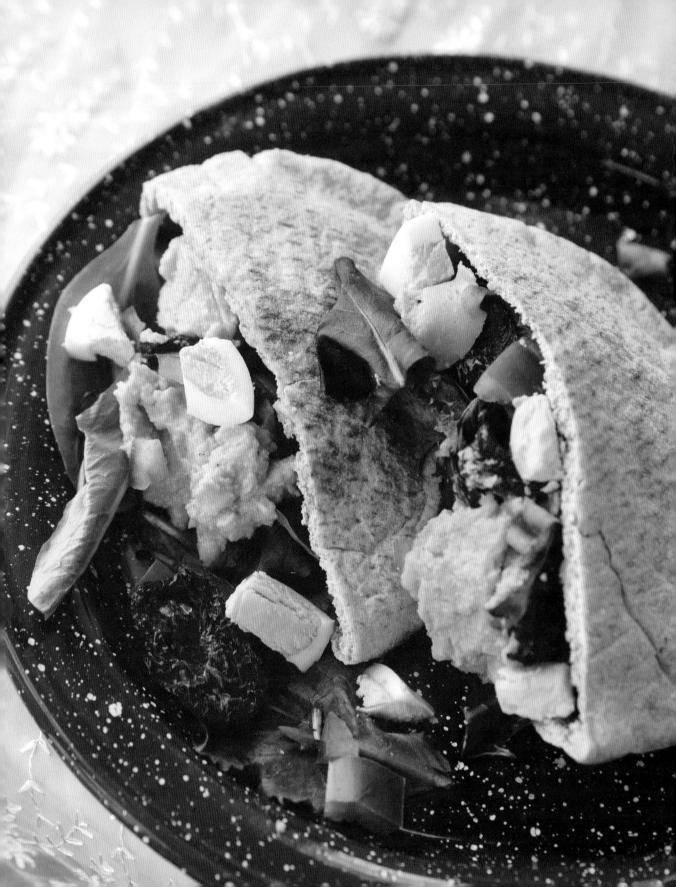

Tomato, Spinach, Egg 'n' Feta Never Tasted Betta Wrap

heart | power2 | can | preg | bones | slim | bloat | skin | stress | mood

If you want a scrumptious, satiating breakfast that will tide you over until lunchtime, energize you, and rejuvenate your skin (and who doesn't?), this will become your go-to meal. Although this nutrient-packed wrap is easy to make, we make it in advance and wrap it in foil in the fridge so that we can grab it on the go.

Yields 4 pita wraps

1. Preheat oven to 350°F.

2. Heat canola oil in a medium pan. Crack eggs in a bowl, add pepper and salt (if using), and whisk. Pour in pan and scramble.

3. Place pitas on a large oven tray, with space between each pita. Divide eggs into four portions and place them in a strip across the middle of each pita.

4. Add tomatoes, feta, and a handful of spinach. Wrap each like a burrito.

5. Place tray in the oven for 5 minutes.

6. Serve whole or cut in half.

Tip: We use a really large pita from Daily Pita Bread that we cut in half (around the edges) to make two individual wraps, so if you can find these pitas, you would need only two of them in the recipe rather than four smaller ones.

2 teaspoons canola oil

8 egg whites and 4 egg yolks (or the equivalent in Egg Beaters)

¾ teaspoon freshly ground black pepper

4 6-inch oat bran pitas or 6-inch whole wheat wraps

2 large diced tomatoes

4 tablespoons light or fat-free feta cheese

1 (6-ounce) bag spinach leaves

Pinch of salt (optional)

Per serving (using Daily Pita Bread and no added salt): calories 121, total fat 7g, saturated fat 2g, cholesterol 210mg, sodium 363mg, carbohydrates 20g, dietary fiber 3g, sugars 1g, protein 18g
Percent Daily Value: vitamin A 102%, vitamin C 35%, iron 14%, calcium 14%

Zucchini Fritters

heart | can | preg | kid | slim | stress | mood | bones

Sunday mornings were all about our mom making fritters for the family, so for us they are a comfort food. However, no need to feel guilty indulging in these for breakfast, lunch—or dinner! These good-size fritters will warm your insides and give you a mood boost for just about 100 calories each.

Serves 4 (two 4-inch fritters per serving)

2 cups coarsely grated zucchini

½ cup coarsely grated white onion

1 egg

2 tablespoons chopped parsley

1 cup cornmeal

1 teaspoon baking powder

¼ teaspoon fresh cracked pepper

2 teaspoons canola oil, divided

Honey, maple syrup, or applesauce for serving

Pinch of salt (optional)

1. Preheat the oven to 200°F.

2. Place the grated zucchini over 3 layers of paper towels in a thin layer. Let sit for at least 30 minutes to lose some excess moisture. (Make sure the grated onion sits as well, for at least 5 minutes before using, to activate its powerful phytonutrient compounds.)

3. After 30 minutes, change the paper towel for new sheets and squeeze the zucchini a little to lose more moisture.

4. In a bowl, whisk together the egg, parsley, and salt (if using). Add the zucchini, onion, cornmeal, baking powder, and pepper. Stir well to combine. The batter will be thick and chunky. Let rest 10 minutes.

5. Add 1 teaspoon of oil to a large nonstick pan over medium heat. When the pan is hot, drop in a scant ⅓ cup of the batter, flattening it into a 4-inch fritter. Cook for 2 to 3 minutes or until the top of the fritter looks slightly bubbly and dry. Turn and cook for another 2 to 3 minutes on the other side. Use the remaining teaspoon of oil as necessary to cook the remaining fritters.

6. Keep fritters warm in the 200°F oven until all are cooked. Serve with a little honey, maple syrup, or applesauce.

Per serving (without salt): calories 216, total fat 4g, saturated fat 1g, cholesterol 53mg, sodium 152mg, carbohydrates 39g, dietary fiber 4g, sugars 4g, protein 6g
Percent Daily Value: vitamin A 10%, vitamin C 36%, iron 17%, calcium 10%

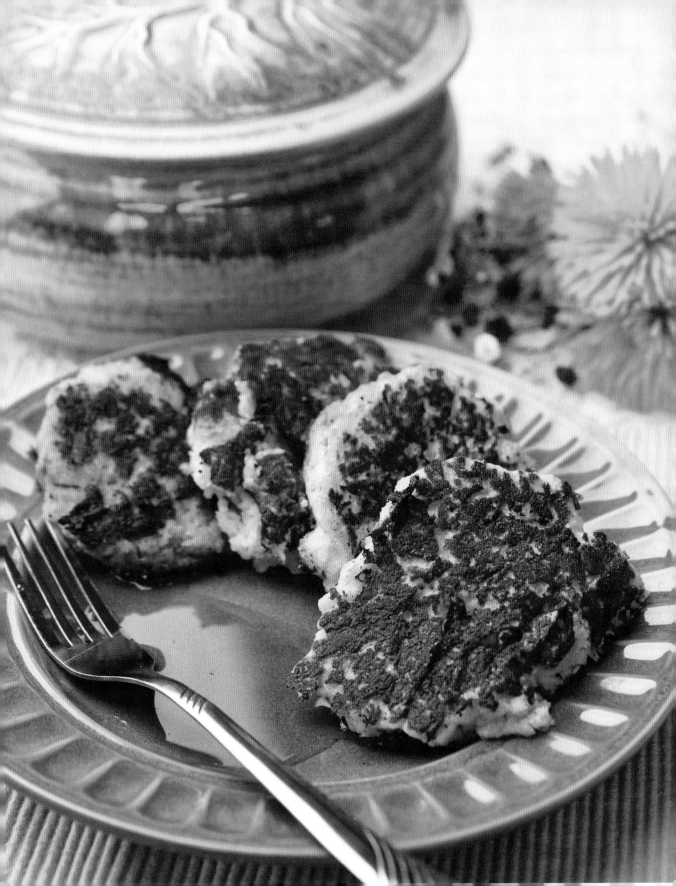

Artichoke Hummus

heart | can | bones | bloat

This variation on traditional hummus is a party pleaser. It's lower in calories than traditional all-chickpea hummus, yet has that delicious, hearty texture that you find in the original Middle Eastern hummus. Unlike many other dips and spreads that are creamy and clog your arteries, this one is good for your heart. We love to pack this in kids' lunch boxes with baby carrots for dipping—such a great way for kids to get extra veggies!

Serves 16 (2 tablespoons per serving)

1 cup canned artichoke hearts, drained

¼ cup fat-free unsalted vegetable broth

¼ cup fat-free plain yogurt

1 tablespoon lemon juice

1½ teaspoons crushed garlic

½ teaspoon dried chives

¼ teaspoon freshly ground black pepper

¼ teaspoon ground cumin

¼ teaspoon paprika

1 (15-ounce) can low-sodium chickpeas (garbanzos), drained and rinsed

1. Put all ingredients except chickpeas into a blender. Blend until uniform.

2. Use a potato masher or a fork to thoroughly mash chickpeas in a bowl. Transfer into blender. Puree until smooth.

3. For best flavor, cover and refrigerate for several hours before serving. Serve with pita chips, crudités, or rice crackers.

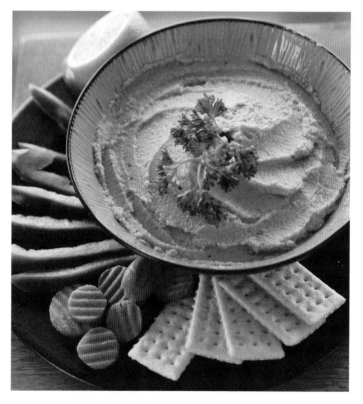

Per serving: calories 36, total fat 0g, saturated fat 0g, sodium 76mg, carbohydrates 7g, dietary fiber 3g, sugars 1g, protein 2g
Percent Daily Value: vitamin A 1%, vitamin C 5%, calcium 2%, iron 2%

Cauliflower Ceviche

heart | can | bones | preg | skin | kid | slim | bloat | stress | mood | detox

We love that you don't have to handle raw meat or seafood to make this tasty ceviche! This unique twist on the traditional ceviche is light and refreshing, and the acid (lime juice) "cooks" the cauliflower. It can be served as an appetizer, a light meal, or a snack. Our recipe calls for corn tortillas, but it works well with baked chips or toasted pita as well.

Serves 4 (1½ cups per serving)

1. Preheat oven to 350°F and place tortillas on baking sheet. Bake for 10 minutes or until crispy.

2. Add lime juice to cauliflower; let it marinate for 15 minutes.

3. Stir onions and cilantro, then tomatoes, into the cauliflower mixture. Toss with remaining ingredients.

4. Enjoy with chips, or place 1 cup of ceviche on your tostada.

> Mangos not only add a hefty dose of vitamin C, vitamin A, and fiber, but they also contain potent phenolics such as ellagic acid and gallotannin, and one specific to mangos—mangiferin. These antioxidants possess powerful anti-inflammatory capabilities (hello, healthier skin!) and anti-cancer qualities that help to boost the body's immune system as well as provide cardiovascular protection.

4 (4-inch-diameter) corn tortillas

Juice of 2 limes

½ small head fresh cauliflower, chopped

2 tablespoons diced onions

½ cup chopped cilantro

1½ tomatoes, diced

1 tablespoon diced green jalapeño

1 mango, in ½-inch cubes

½ teaspoon chipotle seasoning (optional)

Salt to taste (optional)

Per serving (ceviche only, without salt): calories 70, total fat 0g, saturated fat 0g, sodium 42mg, carbohydrates 20g, dietary fiber 5g, sugars 13g, protein 3g
Percent Daily Value: vitamin A 19%, vitamin C 143%, calcium 4%, iron 5%

Carrot Zucchini Muffins

kid | slim | full | skin | detox | preg | can | stress | mood

These juicy nuggets taste like dessert but give you nearly half your daily quota of vitamin A while providing iron, calcium, vitamin C, and fiber to boot. Have one of these and you'll never miss the artery-clogging fat or calories of a store-bought muffin! And if you have kids, serve these and they'll never complain about having to eat their veggies. Plus, they'll get most of the important nutrients that the majority of kids fall short of.

Yields 12 muffins

Cooking spray

1 cup white flour

½ cup whole wheat flour

1 teaspoon baking powder

¼ teaspoon baking soda

¾ cup brown sugar

2 eggs, beaten

1½ cups shredded carrot

1½ cups shredded zucchini

½ teaspoon fresh grated ginger

1 cup shredded granny smith apple

1. Preheat oven to 350°F. Grease a 12-cup muffin pan with cooking spray.

2. In a large bowl mix together dry ingredients: flours, baking powder, baking soda, and brown sugar.

3. In another bowl mix together wet ingredients: eggs, carrot, zucchini, ginger, and apple.

4. Combine the contents of the two bowls and mix until uniform in texture. Pour ⅓ cup of batter into each muffin cup.

5. Bake until muffins are firm to the touch and slightly brown on the edges. Allow to cool for five minutes before removing from muffin tin. Leaving the muffins in the pan for longer could result in soggy muffins. Once muffins have cooled to room temperature (about 30 minutes), they can be wrapped in plastic wrap or an airtight container and refrigerated.

Note: Allow muffins to completely cool before wrapping to prevent them from becoming soggy.

Per serving: calories 132, total fat 1g, saturated fat 0g, cholesterol 35mg, sodium 93mg, carbohydrates 28g, dietary fiber 2g, sugars 15g, protein 3g
Percent Daily Value: vitamin A 47%, vitamin C 9%, iron 6%, calcium 5%

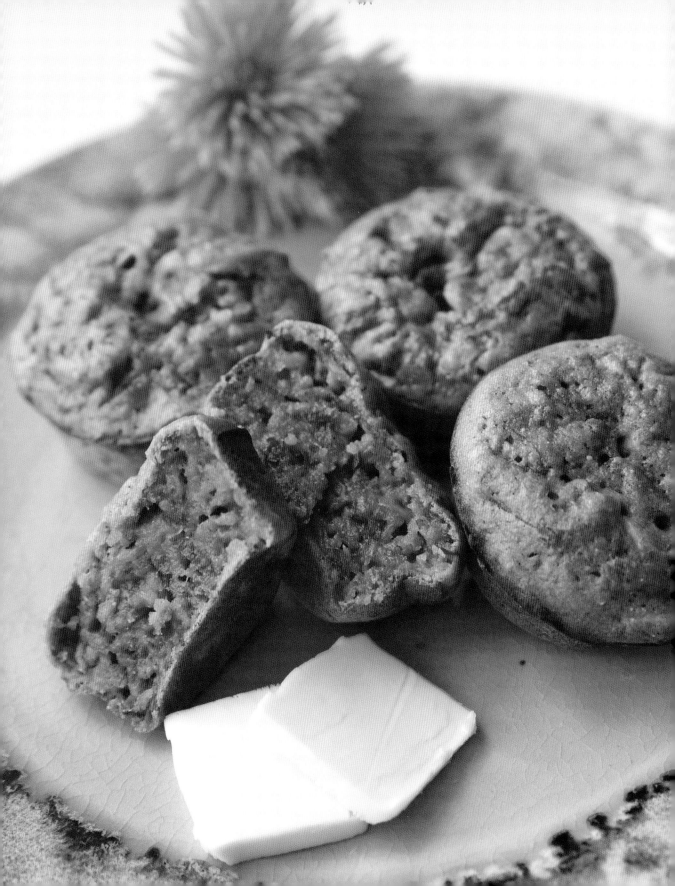

Coco Sweet Potatoes with Mango Salsa

heart | preg | can | kid | bones | bloat | skin | energy | mood | stress | full

This dish is inspired by a coconut-crusted chicken with a mango salsa. If you're like us, you may love the coconut-crusted sweet potato slices so much on their own that you feel they don't even need the mango salsa. This is a dish you can really sink your teeth into, and it will make you happy—even before all of the sweet potato's mood-boosting nutrients make their way into your body.

Serves 4 (3 ounces salsa and 4 potato slices per serving)

FOR THE SALSA

1 small mango, diced (about 1¼ cup)

¼ cup diced green bell pepper (approximately ⅓ pepper)

2 tablespoons diced red onion

½ small jalapeño, seeded, ribs removed, and diced (about 1 tablespoon)

1 teaspoon chopped cilantro

¼ teaspoon ground cumin

½ tablespoon rice or white wine vinegar

¼ teaspoon salt

Freshly ground black pepper to taste

FOR THE SWEET POTATOES

2 large sweet potatoes (approximately 2-inch diameter), peeled and sliced lengthwise ¼ inch thick (about 2 cups sliced potatoes)

1 tablespoon cornstarch

1 tablespoon pumpkin pie spice

¼ teaspoon cayenne

Salt to taste

1 egg white, whisked

¼ cup shredded coconut

Cooking spray

1. Preheat the oven to 350°F.

2. Line two large baking sheets with parchment paper.

3. In a bowl, gently mix together the mango, bell pepper, onion, jalapeño, cilantro, cumin, vinegar, and salt and pepper. Cover and chill in the refrigerator.

4. Place the sweet potato slices in a large bowl. Combine the cornstarch, pumpkin pie spice, cayenne, and salt. Mix together and add to the sweet potatoes and toss well to coat. Add the egg white and toss until the slices are evenly moistened. Sprinkle the coconut over the sweet potatoes and toss again. The coconut will be clumpy, sparingly covering the slices.

5. Place the sweet potatoes on the baking sheet in a single layer. Spread the coconut that is left at the bottom of the bowl on any potato slices that seem like they need more. Spray with a light coating of cooking spray and roast until the potatoes are just tender, about 20 to 25 minutes.

6. Top the potatoes with mango salsa and serve.

Note: After chopping the onions, let them sit for at least 5 minutes before cooking to activate their powerful phytonutrient compounds.

Tip: No fresh mango? You can swap 4 ounces (about ¾ cup) of frozen mango that has been thawed and cubed.

Tip: When cutting the sweet potato, make your first slice lengthwise, then roll the potato over so the cut edge becomes a flat surface against the board. This stabilizes the potato against rolling. Use a sharp knife and take your time making the slices.

Per serving: calories 147, total fat 4g, saturated fat 3g, cholesterol 0mg, sodium 199mg, carbohydrates 27g, dietary fiber 4g, sugars 11g, protein 3g
Percent Daily Value: vitamin A 194%, vitamin C 41%, iron 6%, calcium 3%

Corn and Bean Salsa

full | bones | skin | heart | can | kid | preg | stress | mood | energy

This salsa makes a scrumptious dip that you'll want to keep in your fridge for when snack time rolls around. Dip some carrots in it or spread it on whole grain corn tortillas; you'll get a nice boost of satiating protein and fiber that will keep your blood sugar on an even keel and prevent energy crashes and mood swings. And if dinner rolls around and you're short on flavor (and veggies!), use this to top your favorite chicken or fish dish.

Serves 6 (½ cup per serving)

Mix all ingredients and chill for 2 hours.

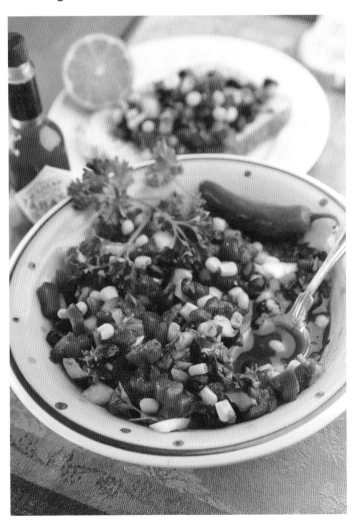

1 cup chopped tomatoes

¾ cup chopped onion

½ cup canned low-sodium black beans

½ cup frozen corn kernels, thawed

2 tablespoons fresh lime juice

2 teaspoons finely chopped parsley

2 tablespoons chopped green bell pepper

1 tablespoon chopped jalapeño

¼ teaspoon freshly ground black pepper

½ teaspoon hot sauce (optional)

Salt to taste (optional)

Per serving (without optional salt): calories 46, total fat 0g, saturated fat 0g, cholesterol 0mg, sodium 14mg, carbohydrates 10g, dietary fiber 2g, sugars 2g, protein 2g
Percent Daily Value: vitamin A 6%, vitamin C 19%, calcium 1%, iron 3%

Curried Sweet Potato and Apple Salad

heart | preg | can | kid | bones | bloat | skin | energy | mood | stress

You can bake the potatoes in the oven or cook them in the microwave. Either way, be sure not to overcook them, as you want diced potatoes to remain intact when you toss the salad. The amount of sugar you will need for the dressing will depend on how "sweet" your sweet potatoes are. This dish is delicious when served immediately, but the flavors marry even more and become more intense when refrigerated overnight. You'll enjoy this dish as much as your kids do!

Serves 6 (generous ½ cup per serving)

2 tablespoons finely chopped onion

1 tablespoon canola oil

1 teaspoon curry powder

¼ teaspoon ground cinnamon

¼ teaspoon ground cardamom

2 tablespoons fresh orange juice

1 tablespoon white wine vinegar

1 tablespoon sugar, or to taste

1 cup tart apple, cut into ½-inch dice

2 cups cooked, peeled sweet potatoes, cut into ½-inch dice

¼ cup raisins

¼ cup coarsely chopped pistachios

1. Chop onions and let them sit for at least 5 minutes before cooking to activate their powerful phytonutrient compounds.

2. Meanwhile, in a large bowl, stir together the oil, curry powder, cinnamon, and cardamom. Stir in the orange juice, vinegar, and sugar until smooth. Add the apples and onion; toss to combine.

3. Add the sweet potatoes, raisins, and pistachios; toss to combine.

4. Serve chilled or at room temperature.

Apples work magic on bad cholesterol. They raise your good cholesterol and lower your bad cholesterol, so they help to lower your risk of heart disease. They also reduce your risk of cancer.

Per serving: calories 177, total fat 5g, saturated fat 1g, cholesterol 0mg, sodium 31mg, carbohydrates 32g, dietary fiber 4g, sugars 15g, protein 3g
Percent Daily Value: vitamin A 345%, vitamin C 29%, iron 7%, calcium 4%

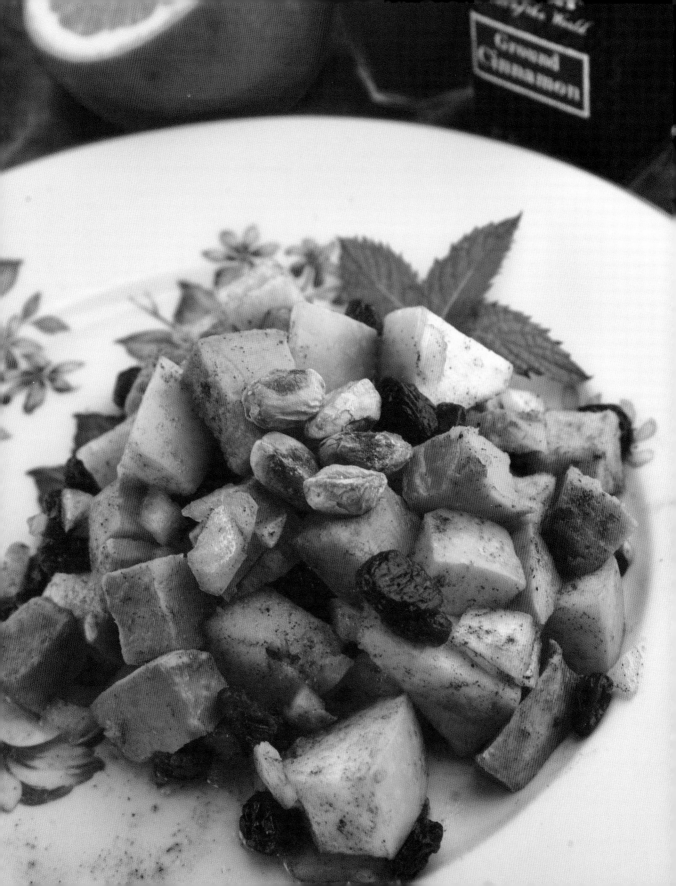

Creamy Spinach Dip

heart | can | preg | bones | bloat | skin | stress | mood

This rich and smooth-tasting dip hits the spot. The water chestnuts add a unique twist and wonderful texture but few calories. Dunk toasted pita, veggies, or baked chips and indulge! You'll fight the blues and beat the bloat all in one swoop.

Serves 16 (2 tablespoons per serving)

1 tablespoon chopped shallot or onion

1 (5-ounce) can water chestnuts, drained

½ cup reduced-fat Neufchâtel cream cheese

½ cup no-salt-added 1% cottage cheese

¼ cup nonfat Greek yogurt

1 tablespoon lemon juice

½ teaspoon freshly ground black pepper

6 ounces fresh baby spinach

2 tablespoons chopped fresh chives or dried chives

1. In a food processor or blender, coarsely chop the shallots and water chestnuts.

2. Add cream cheese, cottage cheese, yogurt, lemon juice, and pepper. Blend until fairly smooth.

3. Add washed, fresh spinach and chopped chives and blend again.

4. Once dip is nice and creamy, with a uniform light green color, place in refrigerator and enjoy in about 1 hour.

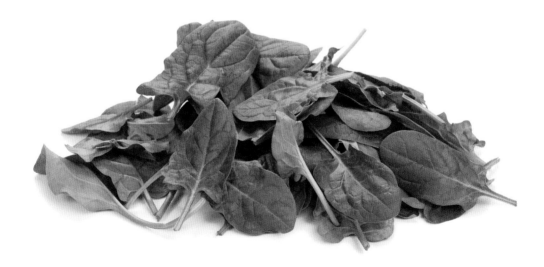

Per serving: calories 45, total fat 1g, saturated fat 1g, cholesterol 4mg, sodium 48mg, carbohydrates 6g, dietary fiber 0g, sugar 1g, protein 2g
Percent Daily Value: vitamin A 21%, vitamin C 11%, calcium 4%, iron 3%

Fig and Olive Tapenade

heart | can | bones | skin

Serve this on whole wheat pita or with crostini and you'll fig'n flip. In fact, your heart may just skip a beat because this heart-healthy, cancer-fighting, bone-boosting tapenade is so flavorful that you could even use it as a delightful sandwich spread or a crudité dip. You'll never have trouble getting your veggie servings again, as it'll be hard to stop dipping. The figs add a fruity hint and creamy texture that is divine.

Serves 13 (2 tablespoons per serving)

1. Place everything but olive oil in a food processor. Pulse until smooth.

2. While the food processor is running, slowly add oil. You are creating an emulsion like a good Caesar salad dressing by adding oil in a slow, thin, and steady stream so that it incorporates and won't separate out.

3. Transfer to a serving bowl or storage jar. You will have about 1⅔ cups. This tapenade will last in the refrigerator for at least a week.

1 cup pitted black olives

1 cup stemmed and quartered fresh figs (brown Turkish or Mission)

2 cloves garlic

1 tablespoon balsamic vinegar

1 teaspoon rosemary

1 teaspoon thyme

Pepper to taste

1 tablespoon extra-virgin olive oil

Salt to taste (optional)

Figs are known for their fiber content: They have 5 grams of fiber in 3 to 5 figs! They also provide more calcium, more potassium, and more iron than many other common fruits and contain no fat, cholesterol, or sodium.

Per serving (without salt to taste): calories 41, total fat 2g, saturated fat 0g, cholesterol 0mg, sodium 89mg, carbohydrates 6g, dietary fiber 1g, sugars 4g, protein 0g
Percent Daily Value: vitamin A 2%, vitamin C 1%, calcium 2%, iron 3%

Garlic and Herb Potato Stacks

heart | preg | can | kid | skin | energy | full | stress | mood

These adorable spud stacks are not only bursting with flavor but really fun to eat. We've served them as hors d'oeuvres and, beware, make extras, because these will get snatched up fast!

Makes 12 servings

Cooking spray

1 pound Yukon gold potatoes (about 2-inch diameter)

¾ pound redskin potatoes

½ cup shredded low-fat Jarlsberg cheese

¼ cup shredded low-fat smoked Gruyère cheese

2 tablespoons extra-virgin olive oil

1 tablespoon spicy brown mustard

1½ teaspoons dried dill

¾ teaspoon McCormick Smokehouse Pepper (or black pepper)

½ teaspoon sea salt

4 cloves garlic, minced

1. Preheat oven to 400°F. Spray 12 muffin cups with cooking spray.

2. In a large bowl, whisk oil and mustard; add dill, pepper, sea salt, and garlic. Mix in cheeses.

3. Cut potatoes into very thin slices, discarding rounded ends. Place in a large bowl with cheese mixture. Mix well with your hands, separating potato slices so that all are as evenly coated with mixture as possible.

4. Stack slices in prepared muffin cups. Scrape bowl to remove all cheese mixture and spoon over potatoes.

5. Bake for 20 minutes, then tent with foil and bake for 20 to 25 minutes more, or until potatoes are tender when pierced with a sharp knife.

6. Serve warm.

Per serving: calories 82, total fat 3g, saturated fat 1g, cholesterol 2mg, sodium 141mg, carbohydrates 12g, dietary fiber 1g, sugars 1g, protein 3g
Percent Daily Value: vitamin A 0%, vitamin C 17%, calcium 6%, iron 4%

Green Pea Hummus

heart | can | kid | bones | bloat | skin | energy | stress | mood

This pea hummus has a delightful sweetness and is great served with whole grain pita for dipping. It's a refreshing and unique alternative to your standard savory chickpea hummus, and Tammy's daughters love it. Our favorite part, aside from the sweet twist, is that it gives us an energy boost while it battles bloat—and it's pretty simple to make, to boot!

Serves 6 (2 ounces per serving)

1. Following the package instruction, steam the peas in the microwave. Alternatively, using a steamer basket in a large saucepan, cook the peas for 6 minutes.

2. While they are still warm, put the peas into the blender along with the rest of the ingredients, except the paprika and pita (see tip). Puree until smooth, about 1 minute. If the hummus is too stiff, add an additional ½ tablespoon of cold water to loosen. The consistency should be very similar to a traditional chickpea hummus.

3. Spread the hummus into a serving bowl and dust with paprika. Cover and chill in the refrigerator for at least 1 hour so the flavors mingle.

4. Remove from the fridge and serve with whole wheat pita. We like to warm the pita on the stove or in the toaster before serving.

Tip: We've found it's best to layer the ingredients into the blender jar in the following order: liquids, spices, garlic, and then the peas on top. This allows the blender to make a slurry with the liquids, which draws the peas down to the blades while keeping the blender from getting clogged.

12 ounces frozen peas, preferably in a microwave steam bag

2 tablespoons tahini (sesame paste)

Juice of 1 lemon

1 tablespoon extra-virgin olive oil

2 dashes of your favorite hot sauce

1 teaspoon ground cumin

¼ teaspoon salt

Freshly ground black pepper to taste

3 garlic cloves, peeled and smashed

¼ teaspoon paprika, for garnish

Whole wheat pita bread, for serving

Per serving: calories 80, total fat 5g, saturated fat 1g, cholesterol 0mg, sodium 140mg, carbohydrates 7g, dietary fiber 2g, sugars 2g, protein 3g
Percent Daily Value: vitamin A 15%, vitamin C 15%, iron 7%, calcium 4%

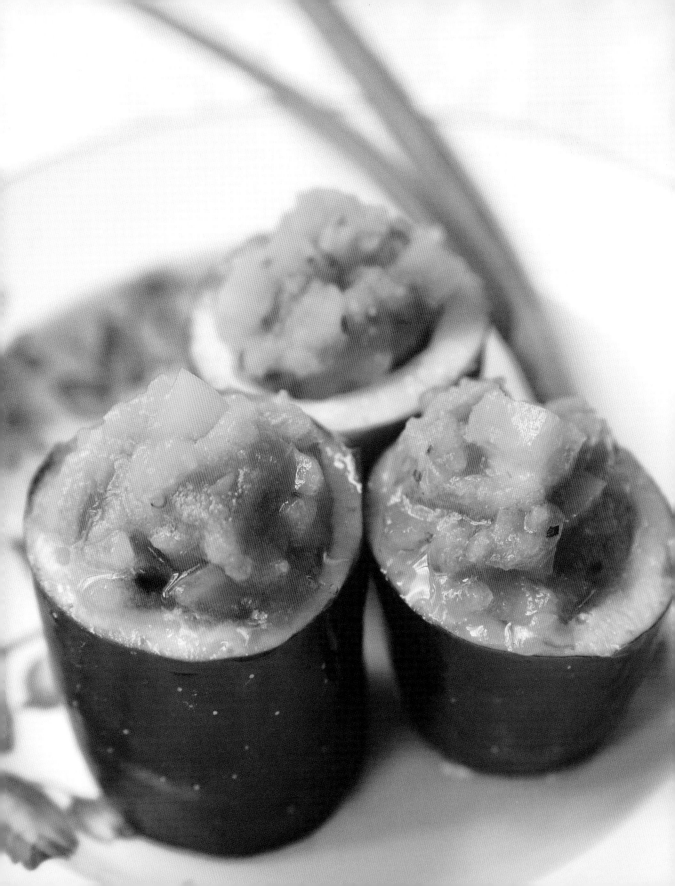

Golden Gazpacho in Petite Cucumber Cradles

heart | can | preg | slim | bloat | skin | stress | mood | bones

This zesty yellow gazpacho is so flavorful that you can forget about asking for seconds—you'll be back for fourth and fifth helpings! We admit, this gazpacho is so scrumptious on its own that we often want more than the appetizer serving and just eat it without the cup. Good thing it's so good for your waistline and will beat the bloat! But do make the cucumber cup, as biting into it makes this even more refreshing . . . and adorable.

Serves 8 as appetizer

1. Place garlic, scallion, tomatoes, and pepper in a food processor and pulse until all vegetables are finely chopped.

2. Stir in the rice vinegar, salt, black pepper, cayenne, and oregano.

3. Cut cucumber into 2-inch lengths and scoop, using a melon baller, to create a mini bowl. Grind a little pepper into each cucumber bowl.

4. Spoon gazpacho into the cucumber bowls and serve.

1 garlic clove

½ scallion

1½ cups cored, seeded, and chopped yellow tomatoes

½ cup diced yellow pepper

1 tablespoon unseasoned rice vinegar

¼ teaspoon kosher salt

¼ teaspoon black pepper

¼ teaspoon cayenne pepper

½ teaspoon dried oregano

1 long or 2 shorter English (hothouse) cucumbers

Fresh grindings of pepper, for serving

Per serving: calories 10, total fat 0g, saturated fat 0g, cholesterol 0mg, sodium 65mg, carbohydrates 2g, dietary fiber 0g, sugars 0g, protein 1g
Percent Daily Value: vitamin A 1%, vitamin C 41%, calcium 1%, iron 1%

Guacamole Stuffed Tomato Poppers

heart | can | power2 | preg | kid | skin | bones | bloat | stress | mood

These poppers are the perfect party pleasers. They are so much fun to eat, and when you pop one into your mouth—a creamy, flavorful explosion! It's hard to believe you get 6 grams of fiber from a serving of these velvety babies. And the fat is coming from the "good for you" fats in the avocado. The toughest part is not eating them all yourself!

Serves 4 (5 tomatoes per serving)

1 garlic clove

20 cherry tomatoes

1 avocado, mashed

Juice of 1 lime

1 tablespoon chopped cilantro (optional)

1 small mango

1. Crush garlic and set aside for 5 minutes to release its health-boosting effect.

2. Wash cherry tomatoes and cut tops off. Carefully cut a sliver off the bottom to help them stand up. Be careful not to cut so deeply as to make an opening on the bottom. Using a melon baller or small spoon, scoop out the insides until hollow.

3. In a bowl mix together mashed avocado, lime juice, garlic, and cilantro.

4. Cut mango into tiny cubes and mix into guacamole.

5. Gently stuff tomatoes with guacamole and serve as a healthy appetizer!

Did you know that one serving of mangos provides 100 percent of your daily vitamin C and 35 percent of your vitamin A, both important antioxidant nutrients? Vitamin C promotes healthy immune function and collagen formation. Vitamin A is important for vision and bone growth.

Per serving: calories 186, total fat 8g, saturated fat 1g, cholesterol 0mg, sodium 17mg, carbohydrates 30g, dietary fiber 6g, sugars 11g, protein 4g
Percent Daily Value: vitamin A 28%, vitamin C 78%, iron 7%, calcium 9%

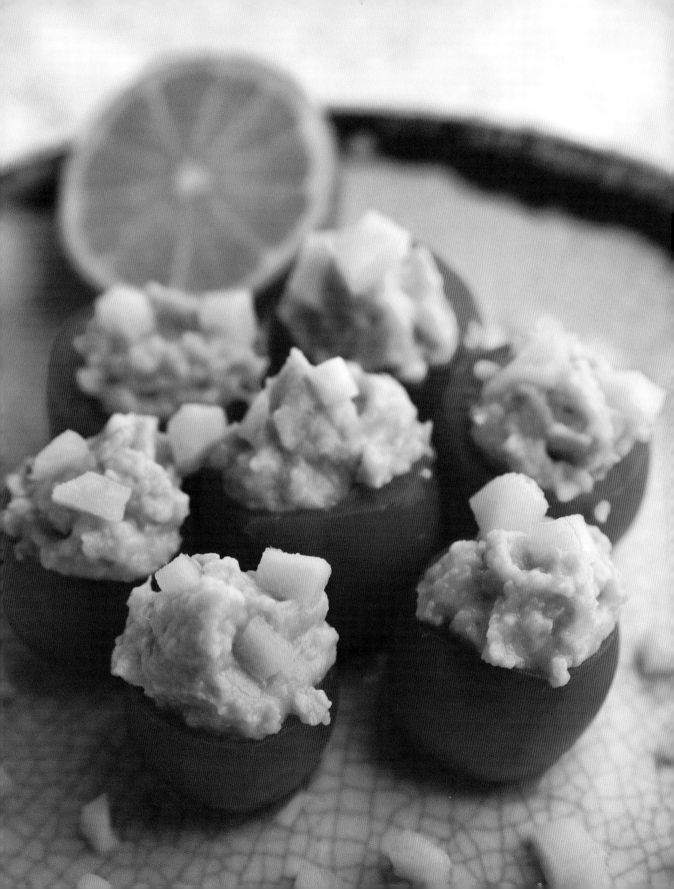

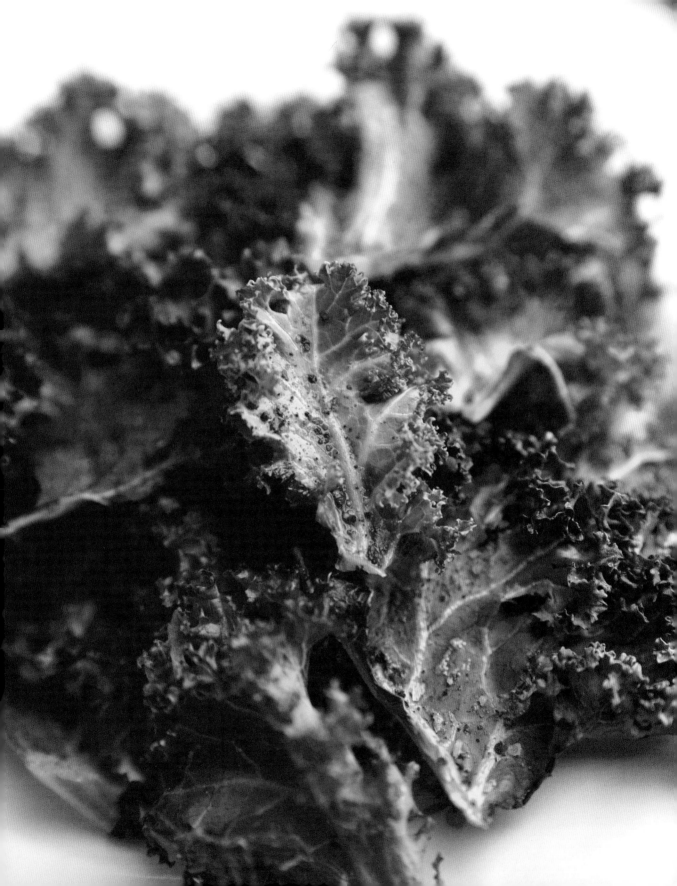

Guilt-Free Kale Chips

heart | can | preg | bones | slim | bloat | skin | stress | mood | kid

These delicious chips are insanely addictive. Feel free to crunch away because, unlike other chips, these allow you to munch without regretting it later. And once you give these to your kids, they'll never be able to tell you they don't like kale.

Serves 6 (⅔ cup per serving)

1. Preheat oven to 350°F. Line two cookie sheets with parchment paper and spray with cooking spray. If you don't have parchment paper, spray the sheets with cooking spray.

2. Cut the kale leaves from the stem, using a knife or kitchen shears, and collect leaves in a large bowl or basin.

3. Wash kale and dry thoroughly, using a towel or salad spinner. Cut leaves into even bite-size pieces, about 2 inches square. Spread kale out on cookie sheets.

4. Spray lightly with cooking spray and sprinkle with seasoning salt and optional spices.

5. Bake until crisp, but not burnt, about 15 minutes.

2 teaspoons olive oil or olive oil spray

1 bunch kale

½ teaspoon seasoned salt such as Lawry's, Morton, or Badia (see sidebar)

Garlic or cayenne pepper (optional)

If you'd prefer to make your own lower-sodium variety of seasoning salt rather than using a commercial blend, mix these ingredients: ¼ cup salt, ½ cup paprika, 1 teaspoon black pepper, 1 teaspoon onion powder, 1 teaspoon garlic powder, and 1 teaspoon celery seed.

For an alternative to Lawry's: 6 tablespoons salt, ½ teaspoon dried thyme leaves, ½ teaspoon marjoram, ½ teaspoon garlic salt or garlic powder, 2¼ teaspoons paprika, ¼ teaspoon curry powder, 1 teaspoon dry mustard, ¼ teaspoon onion powder, ⅛ teaspoon dill weed, ½ teaspoon celery salt. Blend all ingredients together in a blender or food processor until finely ground. Store in a covered container at room temperature.

Per serving (analysis includes 2 teaspoons olive oil): calories 36, total fat 2g, saturated fat 0g, cholesterol 0mg, sodium 127mg, carbohydrates 4g, dietary fiber 1g, sugars 0g, protein 1g
Percent Daily Value: vitamin A 137%, vitamin C 89%, iron 4%, calcium 6%

Holy Fruity Guacamole!

heart | can | preg | kid | skin

If you're a guac fan, you'll love this sweet variation of the traditional guacamole. Thanks to the different textures from the crunchy grapes, the sweet-tart pomegranate arils, and the smooth, creamy avocado and mango, you'll think you died and went to guacamole heaven. The grapes add heart-healthy resveratrol, while the avocados provide nearly 20 vitamins and minerals, and the mango and pomegranate pack vitamin C, fiber, and antioxidants.

Serves 8 (¼ cup per serving)

1 Hass avocado

Juice of 1 lime

½ small shallot, minced

1–2 jalapeño peppers (depending how spicy you like it!), minced

½ cup red grapes, cut in quarters

⅓ cup cubed mango

¼ cup pomegranate seeds

1 tablespoon chopped cilantro

Freshly ground black pepper to taste

1. Peel the avocado, remove pit, and place in a bowl.

2. Mash avocado with a fork until it is smooth with several small chunks.

3. Mix in remaining ingredients and enjoy!

Tip: If you like your guacamole with a little more onion, use the entire small shallot.

Pomegranate arils not only add a delicious crunch, they are also packed with vitamin C and fiber and are a good source of potassium and polyphenol antioxidants, which help neutralize free radicals. This combination makes them great for rejuvenating the skin, while calming your insides and helping to prevent chronic diseases. To save time you can buy ready-to-eat pomegranate arils in the cut-fruit section of most grocery stores.

Per serving: calories 53, total fat 4g, saturated fat 1g, cholesterol 0mg, sodium 3mg, carbohydrates 5g, dietary fiber 2g, sugars 2g, protein 1g
Percent Daily Value: vitamin A 5%, vitamin C 15%, calcium 1%, iron 1%

Muuuhr Muhammara Please

heart | can | preg | slim | bloat | skin | stress | mood

This heavenly dip bursts with flavor. Like traditional muhammara, it's both sweet and fragrant. Muhammara is a common Mediterranean mix used like hummus. But, with its own unique flavor from roasted red peppers and spices and molasses, it also makes a wonderful sandwich spread. You can dip baby carrots in it, like we do, for a great snack!

Yields 28 servings (1 tablespoon per serving)

1. Crush garlic and set aside for 5 minutes to release its health-boosting effect.

2. In a blender or food processor, combine all ingredients: walnuts, roasted red peppers, breadcrumbs, lemon juice, molasses, garlic, cumin, salt, and red pepper flakes. Blend until uniform.

3. Refrigerate for an hour if using as a dip with bread or vegetables. You can also use this as a sauce on kebabs, grilled meats, and fish.

Note: You may also roast your own red peppers and use them instead of the jarred variety.

4 garlic cloves

½ cup walnuts

1 (7-ounce) jar roasted red peppers, drained

⅔ cup breadcrumbs (we use panko, low in sodium and fab!)

2 tablespoons fresh lemon juice

2 tablespoons molasses

1 teaspoon ground cumin

½ teaspoon salt

½ teaspoon red pepper flakes (more if you like it spicy)

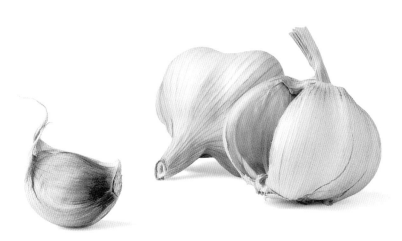

Per serving: calories 23, total fat 1g, saturated fat 0g, cholesterol 0g, sodium 65mg, carbohydrates 1g, dietary fiber <1g, sugars 1g, protein 0g
Percent Daily Value: vitamin A 0%, vitamin C 2%, calcium 1%, iron 1%

I Beg Your Parsnips

heart | can | bones | bloat | stress | mood | detox

We serve these matchstick fries to our families as a super tasty and healthy alternative to french fries. They're fun to eat and packed with flavor. You won't miss the real deal, and neither will your arteries or wardrobe! The pepper gives them plenty of pizzazz—you won't even need the salt!

Serves 2 (½ cup per serving)

Olive oil cooking spray

1 large parsnip (about 9 inches long, 5 ounces), peeled

Cracked black pepper

Salt to taste

1. Preheat oven to 400°F. Line a baking sheet with parchment paper.

2. To make "matchsticks," cut the parsnips into long, thin strips, using a very sharp knife, or a mandoline if you have one. Spray the parsnip sticks with olive oil and lay them on the baking sheet. Lightly sprinkle with cracked pepper on both sides.

3. Bake the fries for about 25 minutes, flipping them over halfway through. They are ready when they are cooked completely, crispy and slightly brown.

4. As you allow them to cool, sprinkle with pepper and salt to taste.

Per serving: calories 50, total fat 0g, saturated fat 0g, cholesterol 0g, sodium 7mg, carbohydrates 12g, dietary fiber 3g, sugars 3, protein 1g
Percent Daily Value: vitamin A 0%, vitamin C 19%, calcium 2%, iron 2%

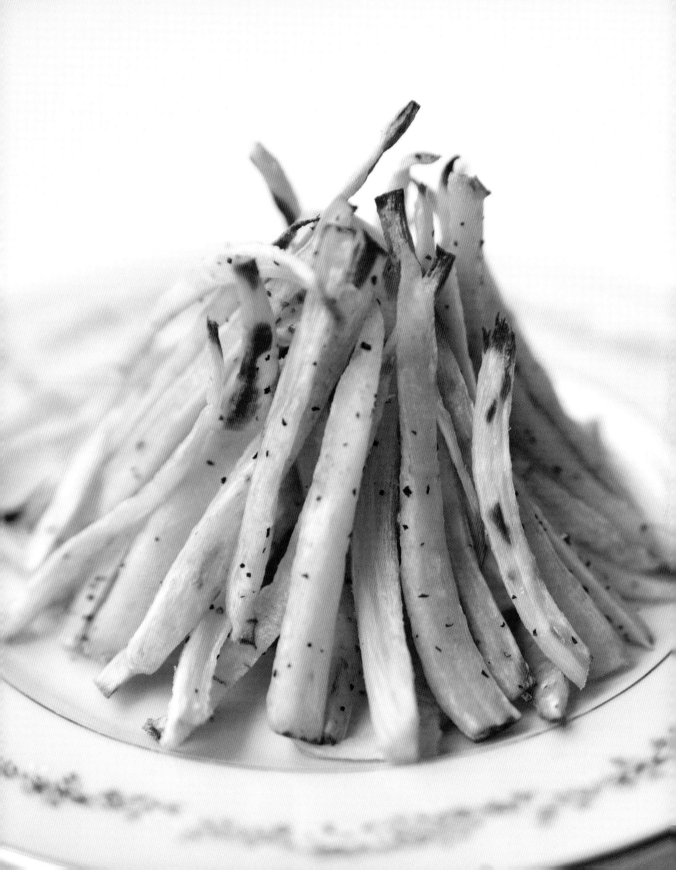

Parmesan Baked Artichoke

heart | can

This dish makes the perfect appetizer for sharing—place it in the center at an intimate dinner party and grab petals as you gab. Plus, it's low in calories, satisfying, and delicious. And unlike most appetizers, it's actually good for your heart, not loaded with artery-clogging fat. It's easy to make, and the simple ingredients allow the wonderful flavor of the artichoke to shine.

Serves 4

1 whole large artichoke

2 tablespoons fresh lemon juice (about 1 lemon)

1 pinch of freshly ground black pepper

4 tablespoons vegetable broth

2 garlic cloves, quartered

1 tablespoon olive oil

2 tablespoons grated Parmesan cheese

1 tablespoon breadcrumbs

1 teaspoon chopped fresh thyme

1. Preheat oven to 425°F.

2. Rinse the artichoke and trim off the sharp points. Cut off the stem so that it will stand upright.

3. Open the artichoke petals as much as possible, being careful to not allow them to snap off.

4. Place the artichoke on a double layer of aluminum foil approximately 12 inches square.

5. In a small bowl mix lemon juice, black pepper, and broth, then drizzle mixture between the petals. Fold up the edges of the aluminum foil so any extra juices stay in the foil.

6. Stuff the garlic quarters between the petals.

7. In a small bowl mix the olive oil, Parmesan, and breadcrumbs together and sprinkle the mixture over the artichoke, letting some fall between the petals.

8. Wrap the artichoke snugly in the aluminum foil and place on a baking sheet.

9. Bake for 55 minutes. Add additional time for an extra-large artichoke.

10. Unwrap the foil enough to expose the artichoke and bake 5 minutes longer to slightly brown the breadcrumbs.

11. Let cool. Garnish with fresh thyme and enjoy.

Per serving: calories 69, total fat 4g, saturated fat 1g, cholesterol 2mg, sodium 141mg, carbohydrates 6g, dietary fiber 2g, sugars 1g, protein 2g
Percent Daily Value: vitamin A 1%, vitamin C 17%, iron 3%, calcium 5%

Pumpkin Cream Cheese Muffins

can | kid | skin | energy | full

These pumpkin muffins are so delicious, we'd choose them over most other desserts. The pumpkin makes these moist and creates a texture like a luxurious cake. They also make a quick grab-on-the-go breakfast that'll provide you with nearly all the vitamin A you need in an entire day!

Serves 12

1. Preheat oven to 350°F.

2. In a large bowl mix pumpkin, applesauce, and egg whites until smooth. In a separate bowl combine the flours, stevia, sugar, baking soda, cinnamon, and nutmeg. Slowly mix the flour mixture into the pumpkin mixture until dry and wet ingredients are blended; do not overmix.

3. For the cream cheese filling: Beat the cheese, sugar, vanilla, egg white, and flour until creamy and smooth.

4. Grease or place papers liners in a 12-cup muffin pan. Fill three-quarters full with batter, then use a clean, wet spoon to hollow out the top center, and fill with 1 tablespoon of cream cheese filling.

5. Bake for about 35 to 40 minutes or until a toothpick inserted in the center comes out clean. Don't overbake, or your muffins will be dry on the edges. Cool and remove from pans. Store in the refrigerator in an airtight container.

1½ cups pureed pumpkin

½ cup unsweetened applesauce

3 egg whites

1 cup all-purpose flour

⅔ cup whole wheat flour

½ cup stevia or other low-calorie/non-nutritive sweetener like Splenda

½ cup granulated sugar

1 teaspoon baking soda

½ teaspoon ground cinnamon

½ teaspoon ground nutmeg

FOR THE CREAM CHEESE FILLING

4 ounces Neufchâtel cheese

⅛ cup granulated sugar

½ teaspoon vanilla extract

1 egg white

½ tablespoon all-purpose flour

Per serving (1 muffin): calories 147, total fat 2g, saturated fat 1g, cholesterol 7mg, sodium 50mg, carbohydrates 28g, dietary fiber 1.5g, sugars 13g, protein 5g
Percent Daily Value: vitamin A 79%, vitamin C 11%, iron 7%, calcium 3%

Ribb—it! Frogs on a Celery-Rib Log

can | slim | bloat | stress | time

This is one of Tammy's top ways to pack a veggie into a kid's lunch box, since it is prepared in just minutes! Celery sticks stay firm in the lunch box, and what makes it a kid-fave is that they love eating the sweet "frogs" (grapes) in their "bed" (low-fat spreadable cheese) on a log (fiber-filled celery). We love that celery fights cancer, bloat, and stress and helps keep you lean.

Serves 2 (3 pieces per serving)

2 celery stalks

1 wedge Laughing Cow Light Creamy Swiss cheese

½ cup (about 36) halved green and/or red grapes

1. Wash celery stalks and cut into 3-inch pieces.

2. Spread cheese in celery ribs, distributing equally.

3. Top with grape halves. If your celery ribs are smaller, you may need to quarter the grapes.

4. Enjoy!

Research has shown that grapes of all colors—red, green, and black—are a natural source of beneficial antioxidants called polyphenols, which may help to defend against aging and disease.

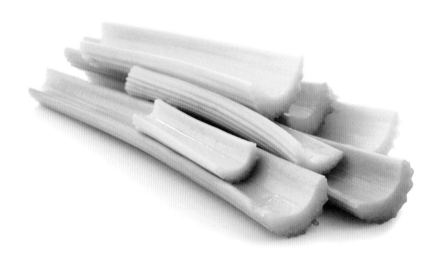

Per serving: calories 22, total fat 2g, saturated fat 1g, cholesterol 5mg, sodium 162mg, carbohydrates 6g, dietary fiber 1g, sugars 5g, protein 2g
Percent Daily Value: vitamin A 4%, vitamin C 6%, calcium 4%, iron 1%

Roasted Turnip Nips

heart | can | bones | bloat | stress | mood | detox | slim

Roasting the turnips mellows their flavor and transforms them into sweet crisps. We love these so much that whenever we eat them, we actually have to try to control ourselves to not eat them all at once, so that we'll be able to share with others. They make a great snack, and each serving is only 25 calories! So if you're trying to lose weight, feel free to indulge in these little nuggets.

Serves 3

1. Preheat oven to 450°F.

2. Trim the ends off the turnips and peel.

3. Cut into 1-inch cubes and place on a parchment paper–lined cookie sheet. Spray with cooking spray.

4. Bake for 20 minutes, turn, and continue roasting another 10 minutes.

5. Remove from oven and toss with black pepper.

2 large (or 4 small) turnips

Olive oil cooking spray

Freshly ground black pepper to taste

Added bonus: These yum-nips are super easy to make!

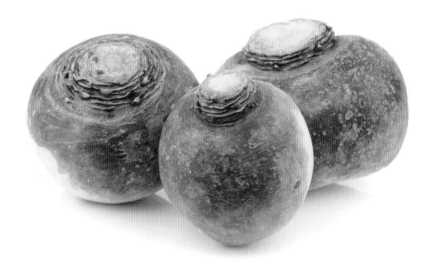

Per serving: calories 25, total fat 0g, saturated fat 0g, cholesterol 0mg, sodium 58mg, carbohydrates 6g, dietary fiber 2g, sugars 3g, protein 1g
Percent Daily Value: vitamin A 0%, vitamin C 30%, calcium 3%, iron 1%

Rockin' Ratatouille

heart | can | bones | skin | full | stress | mood | preg | kid | bloat | detox

This dish is delicious when served either hot or cold. Enjoy with whole wheat crackers, or add whole wheat pasta to make an entire meal. Or you could eat it like we do for a snack, just with a spoon. Your taste buds will feel like they're getting rock star treatment, and if you're trying to lose weight, this is a great choice and you won't feel like you're dieting!

Serves 4 (1 cup per serving)

2–3 garlic cloves, minced

3 tablespoons diced red onion

1 tablespoon olive oil

2–3 medium Roma tomatoes, diced

½ small eggplant, diced

1 teaspoon herbes de Provence (see note)

4 ounces firm tofu, cubed (optional)

1 medium zucchini, sliced

½ medium yellow squash, diced

1 cup sliced mushrooms

2 tablespoons chopped fresh Italian parsley

2 tablespoons pine nuts (optional)

1. In a deep sauté pan or cast-iron skillet, over medium heat, lightly brown garlic and onions in olive oil.

2. Add tomatoes and cook until soft (to release lycopene).

3. Add eggplant and herbes de Provence, and sauté until eggplant softens.

4. If desired, add diced tofu, being careful not to break cubes.

5. Add zucchini, yellow squash, and mushrooms and cook until tender but firm. The dish should have a thin, saucy consistency with colorful cubes of summer vegetables.

6. Add some fresh parsley during the last minute of cooking. Sprinkle with pine nuts for a nice finish.

Note: Herbes de Provence is a mix that may contain any or all of rosemary, thyme, marjoram, basil, bay leaf, summer savory, fennel, chervil, tarragon, and, most distinctively, lavender.

Per serving (with tofu and without pine nuts): calories 90, total fat 5g, saturated fat 1g, cholesterol 1mg, sodium 14mg, carbohydrates 9, dietary fiber 4g, sugars 4g, protein 5g
Percent Daily Value: vitamin A 10%, vitamin C 35%, calcium 9%, iron 7%

Savory Sweet Potato Fries

heart | preg | can | kid | bones | skin | energy | mood | stress | full

Both sweet and savory, these fries are to die for! You get almost twice your daily dose of vitamin A from beta-carotene. If you're a moody kid, or if you're feeling mood dips from extra hormones during pregnancy, or if today is just not your day, this is the perfect "treat" to lift your spirits. It's satisfying and packed with nutrients that boost your energy and your mood. The recipe below includes salt, but you may not need it, so we suggest trying them without the salt, and then adding salt to taste.

Serves 4 (½ cup per serving)

1. Preheat oven to 375°F.

2. Toss all ingredients together, using a large ziplock bag or a bowl.

3. Remove wedges and spread evenly on a large cookie sheet.

4. Bake for 20 minutes, then flip potatoes over and continue cooking until easily pierced with a fork, about 20 minutes more.

2 large sweet potatoes, cut into wedges (about 2 cups)

1 teaspoon basil

1 teaspoon oregano

½ teaspoon thyme

¼ teaspoon sea salt

½ tablespoon garlic powder

½ tablespoon vegetable oil

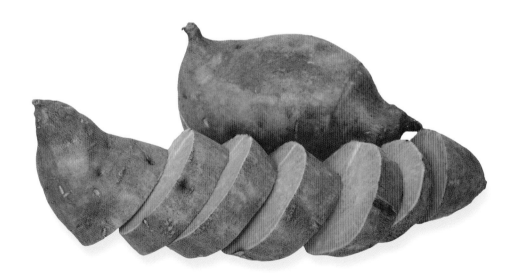

Per serving: calories 71, total fat 2g, saturated fat 0g, cholesterol 0mg, sodium 143mg, carbohydrates 13g, dietary fiber 2g, sugars 3g, protein 1g
Percent Daily Value: vitamin A 185%, vitamin C 2%, iron 2%, calcium 2%

Spinach Squares

heart | can | preg | bones | slim | bloat | skin | full | stress | mood | kid

This dish is inspired by our mom's spinach square dish, which she served frequently when we were kids. It is ultra-satisfying and comforting after a stressful morning or a long afternoon. The protein helps to keep your blood sugar stable and your mood on an even keel—so this dish is great when you want to simply relax and enjoy a great meal. Plus it's a great way to get kids to enjoy spinach . . . everything tastes better with cheese!

Yields 12 squares

Cooking spray

2 teaspoons crushed garlic

3 eggs, beaten

6 tablespoons whole wheat flour

1 (10-ounce) box frozen chopped spinach

2 cups no-salt-added 1% cottage cheese

1 cup skim or part-skim shredded mozzarella

3 tablespoons wheat germ

1. Preheat oven to 350°F. Grease an 8 x 12-inch casserole dish with cooking spray.

2. Crush garlic and let it sit for 5 minutes to increase its health-boosting effect.

3. Mix eggs and flour in a bowl until smooth.

4. Add defrosted spinach, cottage cheese, and mozzarella and mix thoroughly with a whisk or spatula.

5. Pour batter into casserole dish and smooth with spatula, then sprinkle top evenly with wheat germ.

6. Bake for 45 minutes uncovered until sides are golden brown. After it has cooled, cut into squares and serve.

Tip: Turn this "grab-it" snack into a satisfying meal—simply eat two squares!

Per serving (using skim mozzarella): calories 85, total fat 2g, saturated fat 1g, cholesterol 56mg, sodium 111mg, carbohydrates 6g, dietary fiber 2g, sugars 2g, protein 11g
Percent Daily Value: vitamin A 47%, vitamin C 1%, calcium 15%, iron 5%

Stuffed Celery Bites

heart | can | slim | bloat | stress | preg | bones | skin | mood

These make a delicious hors d'oeuvre or lunch box treat. No matter when you eat them, they'll help fight cancer and heart disease and give your skin a glow. Plus, the bean filling is a healthy alternative to the usual cream cheese stuffing for celery.

Serves 4 (about 6 pieces per serving)

1. Chop together the beans, sun-dried tomatoes, and garlic until the mixture is a course puree. Stir in enough of the lemon juice to make the mixture moist. Add the pepper and thyme and stir to combine.

2. Fill the cavity of each of the celery stalks. Lightly dust with chili powder. Cut into 1-inch pieces.

⅓ cup white beans, canned or cooked from dry, drained and rinsed

4 oil-marinated sun-dried tomato halves, chopped

1 large clove garlic, put through garlic press

1–2 teaspoons fresh lemon juice

¼ teaspoon freshly ground black pepper

⅛ teaspoon dried thyme

2–3 large stalks celery, rinsed

Chili powder or paprika (optional)

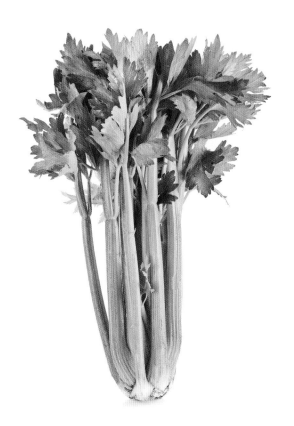

Per serving: calories 36, total fat 1g, saturated fat 0mg, cholesterol 0mg, sodium 43mg, carbohydrate 7g, fiber 2g, sugars 1g, protein 2g
Percent Daily Value: vitamin A 5%, vitamin C 11%, calcium 3%, iron 5%

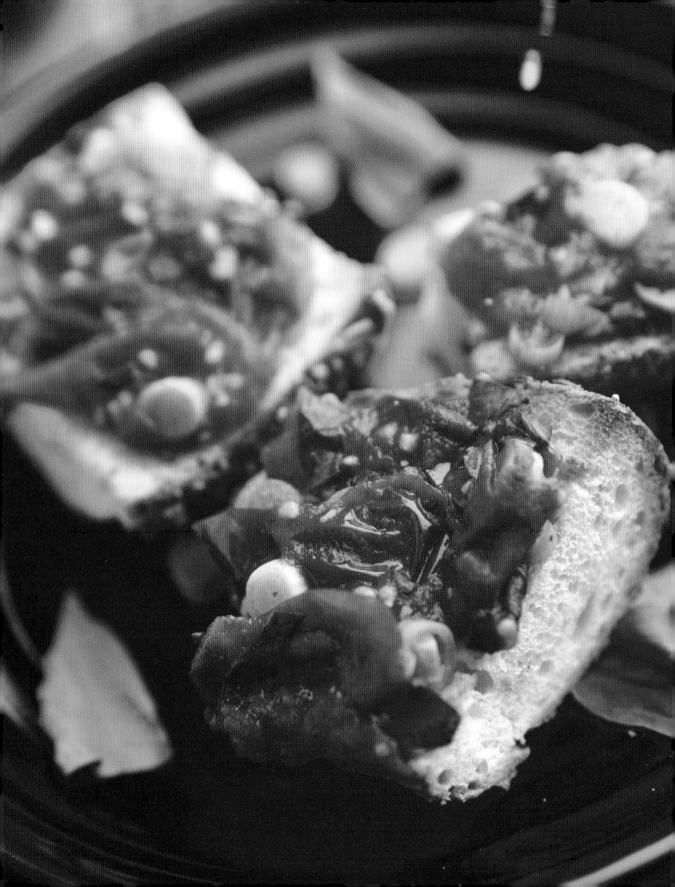

Tomato and Basil Bruschetta

heart | can | preg | bones | bloat | skin | stress | mood

Tammy's husband frequently orders bruschetta at our favorite Italian restaurant, so it inspired us to make our own, which Tammy's husband liked better than the restaurant's! We love that the nutrients it contains helps the entire family to relax and calm down before dinner, while it also helps to make everyone healthy by fighting heart disease and cancer.

Makes 6 servings (1 serving = 4 pieces)

1. Preheat oven to 400°F.

2. Pour 1 tablespoon olive oil into a medium-size (approximately 9 x 12-inch) baking pan and tilt pan until oil covers bottom. Pour in tomatoes and mix so oil coats tomatoes. Lightly grind black pepper over tomatoes and add garlic. Spray olive oil on top and mix until garlic, pepper, and oil are evenly spread throughout.

3. Place in the oven and roast for 20 minutes to allow flavors to mingle as some tomatoes burst.

4. Slice bread into approximately 24 slices, ¼ to ⅓ inch thick. Toast lightly.

5. Remove tomato mixture to a large bowl and add scallions, basil, and salt if wished. Mash tomatoes well, being careful not to get burnt by the hot "insides" of the tomatoes. Mix well and spread on bread.

1 tablespoon extra-virgin olive oil

2 pints grape tomatoes

Freshly ground black pepper

2 teaspoons (approximately 4 cloves) minced garlic

3 sprays olive oil from spray container

1 long French baguette

4 scallions, finely chopped

½ cup finely sliced basil leaves

Salt to taste

Per serving (without salt) of topping: calories 47, total fat 3g, saturated fat 0g, cholesterol 0mg, sodium 7mg, carbohydrates 5g, dietary fiber 2g, sugars 3g, protein 1g
Per serving (without salt) on baguette: calories 139, total fat 3g, saturated fat 0g, cholesterol 0mg, sodium 215mg, carbohydrates 23g, dietary fiber 2g, sugars 4g, protein 5g
Percent Daily Value: vitamin A 22%, vitamin C 26%, calcium 4%, iron 10%

Zucchini Canoes

heart | can | bones | bloat | skin | preg | kid | slim | stress | mood

These canoes are fabulous on-the-go snacks, since you can literally eat a canoe on the go. The bacon and cheese make this veggie taste rich and savory, yet the calories and fat remain low. Tammy's kids love to pretend they're swimming on the "canoe" as they eat it.

Serves 4

2 medium-to-large zucchini

½ tomato, diced

1 small onion, diced

1 clove garlic, minced

½ teaspoon olive oil

¼ teaspoon curry powder

1 tablespoon nonfat Greek yogurt

1 teaspoon chopped or dried chives

¼ teaspoon black pepper

1 tablespoon bacon bits (optional; can be derived from soy or real bacon)

1 teaspoon shredded light cheddar cheese

1. Preheat oven to 400°F.

2. Wash zucchini and scrub the skin with a brush. Slice them in half lengthwise and scoop out the insides to create your boat. Save the insides and chop them, then mix them with the tomato and set aside.

3. Sauté onions and garlic in olive oil until slightly brown and opaque. Then add curry powder and cook for just 30 seconds to prevent it from becoming bitter. Transfer to bowl with zucchini pulp and tomatoes, and mix in yogurt, chives, pepper, and (optional) bacon bits.

4. Stuff the boats with the filling and place them in a lightly greased baking dish. Sprinkle with cheddar cheese and bake for 20 minutes. Take out after the tops are golden brown, and voilà!

Per serving (using soy bacon bits): calories 46, total fat 1g, saturated fat 0g, cholesterol 0mg, sodium 58mg, carbohydrates 7g, dietary fiber 2g, sugars 3g, protein 3g
Percent Daily Value: vitamin A 7%, vitamin C 34%, calcium 4%, iron 3%

Cream of Whatever Soup

heart | can | bones | skin | preg | kid | slim | stress | mood | detox

This soup is super creamy, rich and delicious, and is ideal if you're trying to lose weight. It will fill your stomach for very few calories. Plus, you can use *whatever* vegetable you have around and it still works! Broccoli is one of our favorites, but go with whatever floats your . . . bowl of soup.

Serves 8 (¾ cup per serving)

1. In a medium-size saucepan, on low to medium, heat oil, add onion and garlic, and cook about 6 minutes until golden.

2. Add in frozen vegetable, salt, and pepper, then stir and allow to cook for 5 minutes.

3. Sprinkle flour on top of vegetables and mix thoroughly to evenly distribute the flour.

4. Add 4 cups water, turn heat to high, and bring to a boil.

5. Turn heat down to low and allow soup to simmer for about 20 minutes or until vegetable is tender.

6. Remove from heat and add milk or soy milk.

7. Blend with an immersion blender until smooth.

Note: Allow garlic and onions to sit for 5 minutes after chopping to activate their beneficial compounds.

1 tablespoon vegetable oil

1 cup chopped onion (see note)

4 teaspoons minced garlic

6 cups frozen broccoli or zucchini or cauliflower

1½ teaspoons salt

½ teaspoon black pepper

3 tablespoons whole wheat flour

1 cup low fat milk or soy milk

Per serving: calories 69, total fat 2g, saturated fat 0g, cholesterol 2mg, sodium 356mg, carbohydrates 10g, dietary fiber 2g, sugars 3g, protein 3g
Percent Daily Value: vitamin A 8%, vitamin C 87%, iron 4%, calcium 7%

Cold Cucumber and Avocado Soup

heart | can | preg | kid | skin | bones | bloat | stress | mood | slim

This satisfying, luxurious soup is packed with nutrients. The olive oil is optional; if you have a fruity extra-virgin one, it adds richness. If you just have plain olive oil, don't bother adding the calories, since a generous serving of soup is just 65 calories without it and is definitely fantastic to fill you up and not out. And this soup is just the thing to help you on your way to flawless skin.

Serves 4 (generous 1 cup per serving)

2 cups low-sodium vegetable broth (see page 164)

2 cups peeled, seeded, and cubed cucumber

½ cup ripe avocado (about 1 small)

¼ cup cubed green pepper

¼ cup coarsely sliced scallion

2 tablespoons fresh dill fronds

1 tablespoon extra-virgin olive oil (optional)

1 tablespoon fresh lemon juice

1 clove garlic, minced

1 teaspoon pesto sauce or chopped fresh basil

½ teaspoon ground cumin

¼ teaspoon Worcestershire sauce

½ cup finely diced tomato

Salt to taste

Tabasco sauce or ground red pepper to taste

1. Put the broth, cucumber, avocado, green pepper, scallion, dill, olive oil (if using), lemon juice, garlic, pesto, cumin, and Worcestershire sauce into a blender container (you can also use a food processor, but a blender works best). Cover and blend until fairly smooth.

2. Stir in the tomato. Taste and season with salt and Tabasco sauce or ground red pepper to taste.

> Avocados are a good way to get more lutein in the diet. An ounce of avocado contains 81 micrograms of lutein. Lutein has been shown to be concentrated in the macula of the eye, and research suggests that it may help maintain healthy eyesight as we age.

Per serving (not including salt or Tabasco): calories 95, total fat 7g, saturated fat 1g, cholesterol 0mg, sodium 80mg, carbohydrates 7g, dietary fiber 3g, sugars 3g, protein 2g
Percent Daily Value: vitamin A 18%, vitamin C 38%, iron 6%, calcium 4%

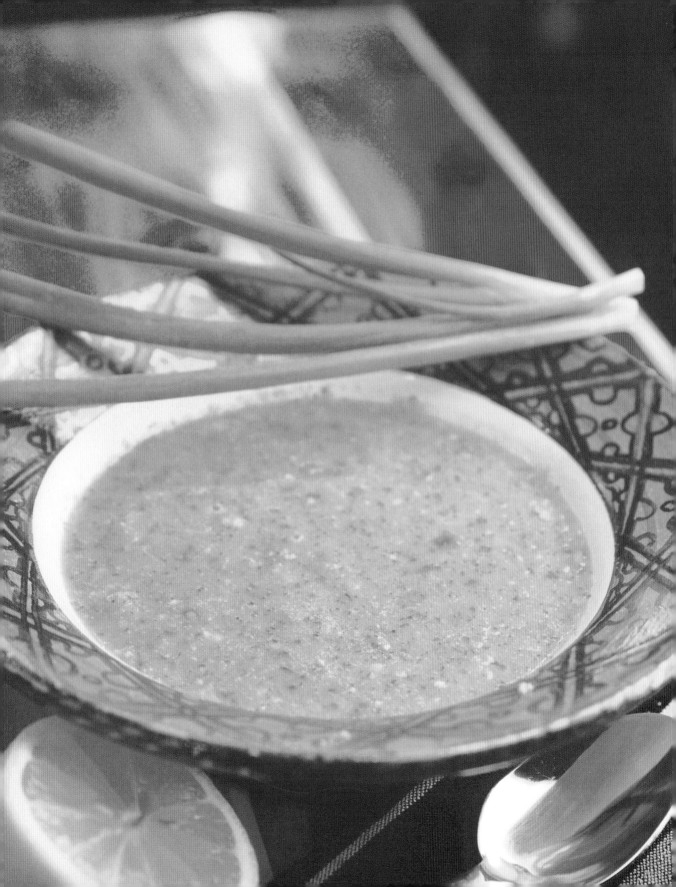

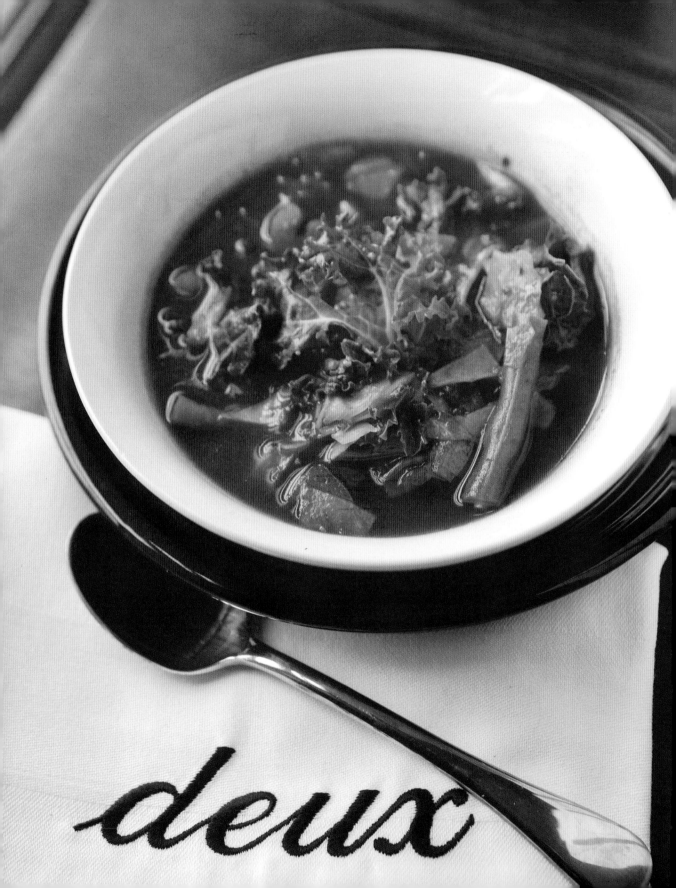

Dieter's Delight Chock Full of Veggies Soup

slim | heart | can | bloat | skin | preg | bones | kid | stress | mood | detox

This soup is so chock full of vegetables and so flavorful, it's perfect for a snack or a meal starter because it fills you up with lots of nutrients. Your taste buds will love it, so you'll want more of this and eat less of the high-calorie stuff. Feel free to leave out any vegetables you don't like and add any fresh or frozen vegetables you do like or have on hand. Just remember that the nutritional information changes when you change ingredients.

Serves 6 (generous 1 cup per serving)

1. Heat the oil over medium-high heat in a 4-quart nonstick pot. Add the cabbage, leek, and green pepper. Cook, stirring, until vegetables are softened, about 3 minutes.

2. Add the broth and marinara sauce; bring to a boil. Add the celery, squash, green beans, okra, bay leaf, oregano, and pepper; return to a boil. Reduce heat and simmer, uncovered, for 30 minutes.

3. Stir in kale and cook for 10 minutes longer. Add salt (if using) and discard the bay leaf.

1 tablespoon olive oil

3 cups shredded cabbage

1 cup sliced leek

½ cup chopped green bell pepper

4 cups low-sodium vegetable broth (see next page)

2 cups low-sodium marinara sauce

1 cup sliced celery

1 cup sliced yellow squash

1 cup cut green beans, fresh or frozen

½ cup sliced okra (optional)

1 bay leaf

½ teaspoon oregano

¼ teaspoon ground black pepper

1 cup coarsely chopped kale (or escarole or spinach or Swiss chard)

Salt to taste (optional)

Per serving (without added salt): calories 89, total fat 4g, saturated fat 1g, cholesterol 0g, sodium 119mg, dietary fiber 5g, sugars 8g, protein 3g
Percent Daily Value: vitamin A 49%, vitamin C 80%, calcium 8%, iron 10%

Vegetable Broth

heart | can | slim | skin | detox | stress | bloat

This very flavorful broth is made by chopping the vegetables into tiny pieces so that there is lots of surface area and the vegetables give more flavor to the broth than if they were just used whole. The broth is quite concentrated, and you can add more water to taste if you want it to be "milder." We freeze this broth in ice cube trays and simply use a few broth cubes to "sauté" veggies as we need them. This makes a tasty and great anti-bloat alternative rather than using oil or butter, cutting the calories and fat; it can be used in our recipes that call for low-sodium broth, or it could be the base of a quick soup when you want to "detox."

Serves 6 (1 cup per serving)

3 medium carrots (12 ounces total), peeled and cut into chunks

3–4 large stalks celery (8 ounces total), peeled and cut into chunks

1 medium leek (5 ounces), white to dark green parts, cut into chunks and well rinsed

1 small turnip (3 ounces), peeled and cut into chunks

1 medium parsnip (3 ounces), peeled and cut into chunks

1 ripe medium tomato (6 ounces), cut into chunks

Small bunch parsley

¼ cup celery leaves

2 cloves garlic, halved

Salt to taste (optional)

1. Process the carrot in a food processor until very finely chopped; place in a 4-quart pot. Repeat with the celery, then the leek, then the turnip and parsnip. Put the tomato, parsley, celery leaves, and garlic in the processor and process until smooth. Add to the pot.

2. Add 6 cups water to the vegetables in the pot. (If you'd like to further dilute the broth, you can add more water.) Place on high heat and bring to a boil. Reduce heat and simmer, uncovered, for 1 hour, stirring occasionally. Strain into a large bowl, pressing the vegetables to release any liquid. Season with salt to taste (if desired).

Note: If you dilute the broth, you will reduce calories and sodium but also other nutrients.

Per serving: calories 65, total fat 0g, cholesterol 0mg, sodium 98mg, carbohydrates 15g, dietary fiber 4g, sugars 6g, protein 2g
Percent Daily Value: vitamin A 206%, vitamin C 31%, calcium 7%, iron 6%

Herbed Pea Soup with Spinach

energy | heart | can | preg | bones | slim | bloat | skin | full | stress | mood

If you've had a tough week, and comfort food and relaxation are calling your name, get your spoon ready! Aside from the delicious flavor of this soup, we love that it provides an incredible long-lasting energy boost and is just the thing to get you through a long day . . . or a tiring week. We make this in advance and save it in the freezer for those days when we need it. It's great to come home and know we can just heat this up and dive in. Although fresh herbs are delightful in this soup, you can substitute dried herbs, just use half as much and add them when you add the peas. Feel free to replace the spinach with turnip greens in this soup.

Serves 4 (generous 1 cup per serving)

1. In a 3-quart saucepan, heat the oil over medium-high heat. Add the leeks and cook, stirring, until softened, about 2 minutes.

2. Add the broth and bring to a boil. Add the peas and rice to the broth and return to a boil. Reduce heat and simmer, uncovered, for 25 minutes or until the rice is fully cooked.

3. Place the soup in a blender container (or use an immersion blender) along with the mint, dill, tarragon, and pepper. Cover and blend until smooth. Return to the saucepan and add the spinach. Cook, stirring occasionally, until spinach is thawed and soup is heated, about 7 minutes. Season with salt (if desired).

1 tablespoon olive oil

1 cup sliced leek, white and light green parts, well rinsed

4 cups low-sodium vegetable broth (see page 164)

1 (10-ounce) box frozen peas

2 tablespoons uncooked long-grain white rice

2 large mint leaves

1 teaspoon fresh dill fronds

½ teaspoon fresh tarragon leaves

¼ teaspoon freshly ground black pepper

1 (10-ounce) box frozen chopped spinach

Salt to taste (optional)

Per serving (without added salt): calories 169, total fat 6g, saturated fat 2g, cholesterol 0mg, sodium 272mg, carbohydrates 23g, dietary fiber 6g, sugars 6g, protein 8g
Percent Daily Value: vitamin A 201%, vitamin C 32%, iron 18%, calcium 12%

Split Pea and Barley Soup

heart | can | kid | bones | bloat | skin | energy | stress | mood | slim | full | detox

This soup is another one that's inspired by the comforting, hearty, and delicious soup our mom makes. The barley adds a wonderful meaty texture, and the great thing about this soup is that you simply throw everything in the pot and let it cook, stirring it on occasion. We like this soup thick and stew-like, so we let it cook for several hours. Then we just sink our teeth in and let the warmth and its nutrients peel away the stress. This soup is also fiber-filled and can clean out the "pipes" if you're feeling bloated from constipation.

Serves 6 (about 1 cup per serving, if prepared thick)

1 cup dried split peas

½ cup pearled barley

3 cups chopped onion

1½ cups chopped celery

2 cups chopped carrots

2 cloves garlic, minced

1 cup frozen mixed veggies (optional)

Salt and pepper to taste

¼ cup chopped fresh dill (optional)

1. Rinse split peas and pearled barley in a strainer.

2. Place all ingredients in a 4-quart pot over medium heat and cook for 2½ to 3 hours, until the split peas are soft and very tender, or dissolved if you prefer. Stir occasionally as the soup thickens, to prevent it from scorching. You may need to add more water if it starts to get too thick for your taste.

3. When soup is almost done, add frozen vegetables, salt, pepper, and dill to taste and allow veggies to cook for 5 to 10 minutes.

Note: If you like yours soupier and less stew-like, add more water as it cooks.

Per serving: calories 125, total fat 0, saturated fat 0g, cholesterol 0mg, sodium 78mg, carbohydrates 26g, dietary fiber 7g, sugars 8g, protein 5g
Percent Daily Value: vitamin A 165%, vitamin C 17%, calcium 7%, iron 6%

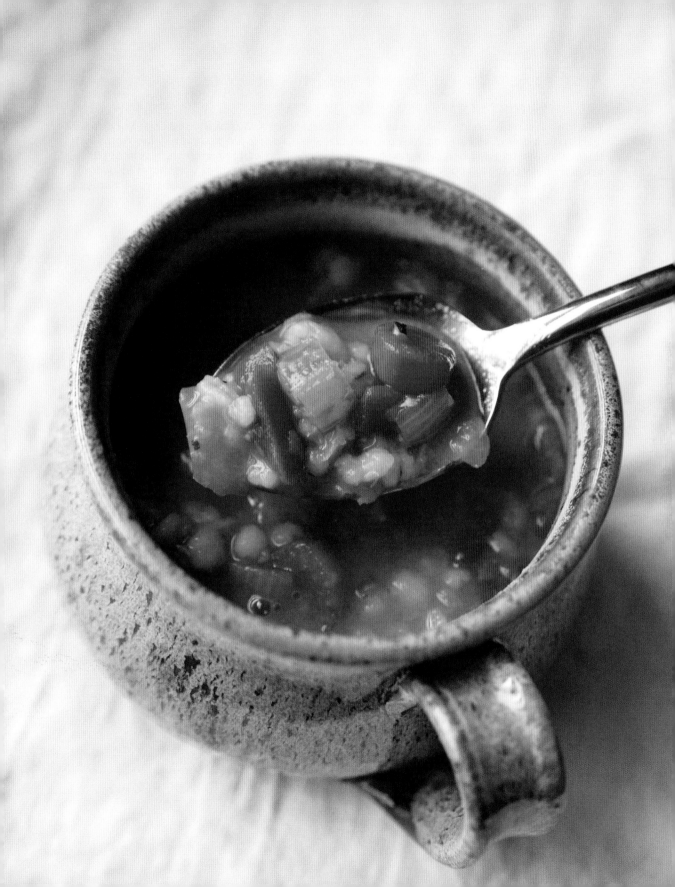

Arugula Salad with Strawberry Rhubarb Vinaigrette

heart | can | preg | kid | skin

This salad is sure to please any dinner guest. Arugula mixed with sweet strawberries, delicate rhubarb vinaigrette, and creamy feta cheese make this salad divine. It's a great way to get kids to eat arugula! And your body will thank you for the hefty dose of antioxidants from the red and green produce that keep you healthy.

Serves 3

½ cup chopped frozen rhubarb

¾ cup chopped frozen strawberries

½ cup coarsely chopped shallots

½ tablespoon sugar

3 tablespoons red wine vinegar

2 tablespoons canola oil

¼ teaspoon Dijon mustard

10 cups arugula

½ cup sliced fresh strawberries

1 ounce feta cheese

¼ cup sliced avocado (optional)

1. In a small saucepan combine rhubarb, strawberries, shallots, sugar, and vinegar. Simmer until soft, about 10 minutes.

2. Allow to cool and then blend with a blender. Strain mixture through a sieve into a medium bowl.

3. Add oil and mustard and mix thoroughly.

4. In a large salad bowl combine the arugula, strawberries, cheese, and dressing. Mix. Top with avocado slices (if desired).

Did you know? California strawberries are packed with essential vitamins, fiber, potassium, and phytonutrients. One serving, about eight strawberries, is an excellent source of vitamin C. In fact, a serving of strawberries is just the skin-dulgence nutrient package your complexion craves for a rejuvenated glow.

Per serving (without optional avocado): calories 187, total fat 11g, saturated fat 2g, cholesterol 8mg, sodium 128mg, carbohydrates 18g, dietary fiber 3g, sugars 8g, protein 4g
Percent Daily Value: vitamin A 40%, vitamin C 87%, iron 11%, calcium 22%

Colorful Crunch Salad with Honey Dijon Vinaigrette

heart | preg | can | bones | kid | bloat | skin | stress | mood | slim

We love to place this salad on a tray in the middle of the dinner table because all of its bright colors make it super enticing. In fact, it's so colorful that one of Tammy's daughters' favorite things to do as she crunches away and enjoys the burst of flavor is count the veggie colors of the rainbow. And it has its perfect complement in the honey Dijon vinaigrette, our favorite low-calorie dressing.

Serves 10 (1 cup salad and 1 ounce dressing per serving)

1. Place raisins in a small bowl of warm water for 5 minutes to plump.

2. Toss tomatoes, cucumbers, peppers, lettuce, and apples in a large bowl. Set aside.

3. Place all dressing ingredients in a bowl and whisk together.

4. When ready to serve, spoon dressing over salad and sprinkle with nuts and raisins.

California raisins are packed with antioxidant protection for heart and colon health. They are a fabulous source of all-natural energy, helping this salad to give you a boost with all of its color. They also add a nice dose of fiber to aid healthy digestion, and potassium for relaxation. The pistachios are rich in potassium and magnesium and are also a good source of B vitamins to really increase nutrients and give you a mood boost.

FOR THE SALAD

⅓ cup golden raisins

⅓ cup California raisins

2 large tomatoes, sliced

2 cucumbers, sliced

1 red bell pepper, roughly chopped

1 green bell pepper, roughly chopped

1 yellow bell pepper, roughly chopped

1 orange bell pepper, roughly chopped

½ head romaine lettuce, washed and torn into bite-size pieces

2 Gala apples, peeled, cored, and diced

½ cup pistachios

FOR THE HONEY DIJON VINAIGRETTE

3 tablespoons lemon juice

3 tablespoons red wine vinegar

1 teaspoon extra-virgin olive oil

1½ teaspoons Dijon mustard

1 teaspoon honey

¼ teaspoon black pepper

⅛ teaspoon dried basil

Dash of salt

Per serving (with 2 tablespoons dressing): calories 131, total fat 4g, saturated fat 0g, cholesterol 0mg, sodium 65mg, carbohydrates 22g, dietary fiber 3g, sugars 13g, protein 3g
Percent Daily Value: vitamin A 72%, vitamin C 183%, calcium 3%, iron 8%

Asian Lettuce Wrap with Hoisin-Ginger Dipping Sauce

heart | can | preg | can | skin | stress | mood | bones

This dish was inspired by one of our favorite vegetable wraps from a local Japanese restaurant. We crave this dish frequently, and it's one of our all-time favorites. We actually love it more than the original inspiration! We really enjoy how the dish bursts with flavors while packing in protein, vitamin E, fiber, magnesium, folate, and niacin from the peanuts.

Serves 8 (1 cup salad and 1 ounce sauce per serving)

FOR THE DRESSING

¼ cup honey

¼ cup rice vinegar

1 tablespoon low-sodium soy sauce

½ teaspoon Asian sesame oil

1 tablespoon peanut butter

½ teaspoon sriracha sauce

1 tablespoon minced fresh ginger

1 large garlic clove, minced

FOR THE SLAW

4 cups (14-ounce bag) prepared shredded coleslaw

1 red bell pepper, diced

2 tablespoons sliced scallions

2 tablespoons chopped fresh mint

½ cup sliced water chestnuts

½ cup unsalted chopped peanuts

2 cups frozen shelled edamame

½ cup chopped fresh cilantro (optional)

FOR THE DIPPING SAUCE

(Makes ½ cup, or eight 1 tablespoon servings)

2 tablespoons hoisin

1 garlic clove, chopped

2 tablespoons brown sugar

2 tablespoons grated ginger

4 teaspoons low-sodium soy sauce

5 teaspoons rice wine vinegar

2 tablespoons chopped cilantro (optional)

1 tablespoon fresh lemon juice (about ½ lemon)

1 tablespoon Asian sesame oil

FOR THE WRAP

8–12 bibb or Boston lettuce leaves

Per serving (without dipping sauce): calories 205, total fat 9g, saturated fat 1g, cholesterol 5mg, sodium 96mg, carbohydrates 24g, dietary fiber 4g, sugars 11g, protein 8g
Percent Daily Value: vitamin A 10%, vitamin C 57%, calcium 6%, iron 10%
Per serving (dipping sauce, 1 tablespoon): calories 38, total fat 2g, saturated fat 0g, cholesterol 0mg, sodium 133mg, carbohydrates 5g, dietary fiber 0g, sugars 4g, protein 0g

1. Prepare the dressing by combining all the ingredients in a mixing bowl with a whisk until well blended. Set aside.

2. Prepare the slaw by combining the coleslaw, red pepper, scallions, fresh mint, water chestnuts, peanuts, edamame, and cilantro (optional) in a large bowl.

3. Prepare the dipping sauce by combining all the ingredients with a whisk until well blended. Set aside.

4. Add the dressing to the slaw (approximately 2 tablespoons of dressing per cup of slaw). Toss well and let stand for 5 minutes.

5. Lay the lettuce leaves out flat, fill each with approximately 1 cup of the dressed slaw mix, and fold the leaf up into a roll.

6. Serve with the hoisin dipping sauce and enjoy.

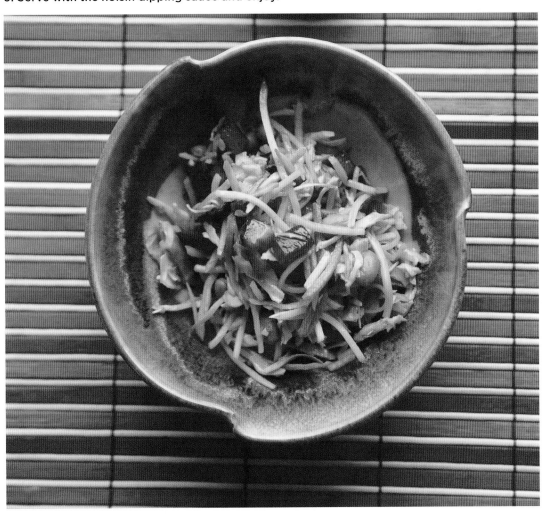

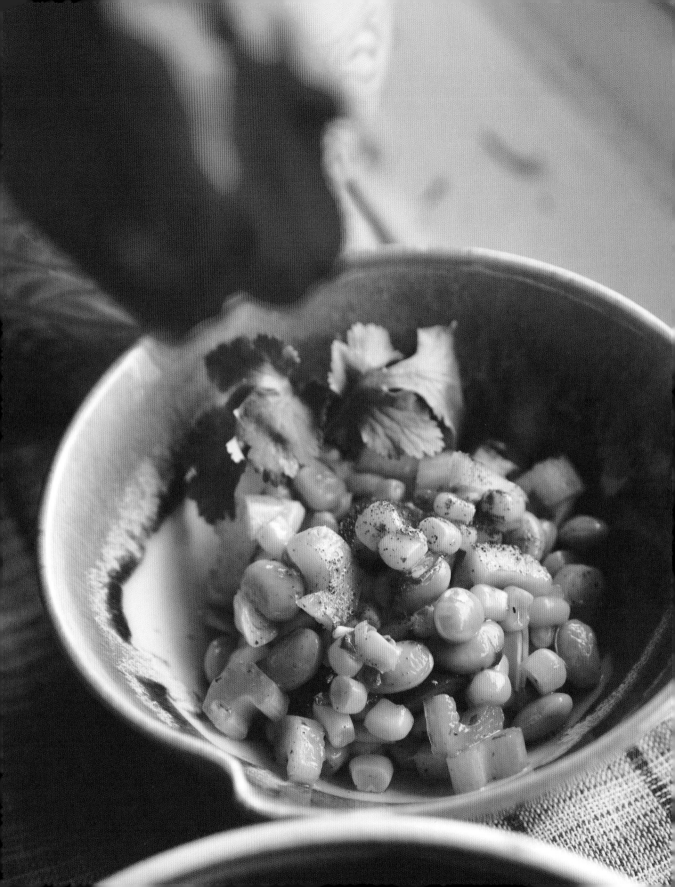

Edamame and Corn Salad

heart | can | kid | preg | stress | mood | bones | skin | energy

Edamame are fresh soybeans and are most commonly available frozen either in the shell or shelled. They make great snacks in the shell, a fun nutritious snack for kids. For cooking it's best to buy the shelled ones, as shelling can be time-consuming. Don't fret if you do not have smoked paprika on hand—the salad is delicious even without it. When we crave this salad, we feel really good about eating it, especially knowing it helps to strengthen our bones.

Serves 6 (generous ⅓ cup per serving)

1. In a small saucepan cook the edamame in boiling water for 5 minutes. Pour into a strainer or colander, drain well, and cool.

2. Place the cooled edamame, corn, celery, olives, onion, and cilantro in a large bowl.

3. Add the vinegar, both oils, Old Bay seasoning, and smoked paprika (if using). Toss to combine.

4. Season with salt to taste if needed.

Note 1: You may choose to use no-salt-added canned corn, or 1 cup of fresh or frozen corn kernels, cooked.

Note 2: If available, use reduced-salt olives, such as Pearls Reduced Salt Large Pitted California Ripe Olives.

1 cup frozen shelled edamame

1 (8-ounce) can corn kernels, drained (see note 1)

½ cup chopped celery

⅓ cup sliced black olives (see note 2)

¼ cup finely chopped red onion

1 tablespoon chopped cilantro

2 tablespoons cider vinegar

1 tablespoon canola oil

1 teaspoon olive oil

1 teaspoon Old Bay seasoning or seasoned salt

⅛ teaspoon smoked paprika (optional)

Salt to taste

Per serving (with no-salt-added canned corn and no additional salt): calories 98, total fat 5g, saturated fat 1g, cholesterol 0mg, sodium 152mg, carbohydrates 11g, dietary fiber 2g, sugars 1g, protein 4g
Percent Daily Value: vitamin A 3%, vitamin C 6%, iron 9%, calcium 4%

Grapefruit, Avocado, and Kale Salad with Pepitas

heart | preg | can | bones | kid | bloat | skin | slim | mood | stress | detox

This light and refreshing tropical green salad makes for the perfect starter. Yet it's so delicious that you may just decide you want to have two servings and make a light lunch. Either way, your skin will get a rejuvenating glow thanks to avocado's anti-inflammatory properties, which will minimize flare-ups and tone skin in combination with the hydrating grapefruit.

Serves 4 (1½ cups per serving)

FOR THE SALAD

1 head lacinato kale

1 grapefruit, peeled, segmented, and chopped small

½ avocado, cubed small

1 tablespoon raw pepitas (pumpkin seeds)

FOR THE DRESSING

1 shallot, minced

1 tablespoon fresh lemon juice

Zest of ½ lemon, grated

1 teaspoon extra-virgin olive oil

Pinch of freshly cracked black pepper

1. Remove the tough stems from the kale leaves. Cut the leaves into bite-size pieces.

2. In a small bowl whisk together the shallot, lemon juice, lemon zest, olive oil, and black pepper.

3. Pour the dressing over the kale, toss to coat the leaves, and let sit for 10 minutes or until the kale begins to wilt.

4. Add grapefruit, avocado, and pumpkin seeds. Toss and serve.

Grapefruit's tangy sweetness pairs well with this salad. Grapefruit is fabulous if you're striving to achieve or maintain a healthy weight, since it's got fiber and a high water content to help you feel full and satisfied. It also will help to prevent cell and tissue damage and the accompanying chronic diseases, thanks to its being an excellent source of vitamin C.

Per serving: calories 120, total fat 7g, saturated fat 1g, cholesterol 0mg, sodium 32mg, carbohydrates 14g, dietary fiber 4g, sugars 3g, protein 4g
Percent Daily Value: vitamin A 216%, vitamin C 166%, iron 11%, calcium 10%

Hickory Broccoli Salad

heart | can | kid | skin | time | power2 | preg | bones | stress | mood | slim

This salad makes a large amount, so it's great for a party or for making in advance on a Sunday to have for several days so you can get your veggies. And as we've learned from serving many guests, everything is better with a touch of bacon. If you're like us and prefer the crunchy soy bacon bits, add them just before serving. It's a great way to cut back on salt, because a little bit adds a lot of flavor. You'll also get a healthy dose of fiber—and this salad is very waistline friendly!

Serves 6 (1 cup per serving)

1. In a small dish soak raisins in warm water for 5 minutes to plump.

2. While the raisins are soaking, make the dressing. Mix the yogurt and mustard until the sauce is homogeneous. Fold in the parsley and the onion and garlic powders.

3. In a large serving bowl, combine the broccoli, tomatoes, mushrooms, bacon bits, and raisins.

4. Pour dressing over the vegetables and toss until they are coated.

Tip: Simply let your frozen broccoli thaw overnight in the fridge. Drain it the next day and use it in this recipe—its wetness will add nice moisture to the salad. You can use raw broccoli if you don't have frozen, although frozen is ideal.

FOR THE SALAD

¼ cup raisins

4 cups frozen, thawed broccoli florets (see tip)

2 cups chopped tomatoes

1 cup sliced mushrooms

4 teaspoons bacon-flavor soy bits (3 slices soy bacon)

FOR THE DRESSING

¾ cup plain fat-free yogurt

1½ tablespoons grainy Dijon mustard

1 tablespoon dried parsley

¼ teaspoon onion powder

⅛ teaspoon garlic powder

Per serving: calories 68, total fat 1g, saturated fat 0g, cholesterol 0mg, sodium 98mg, carbohydrates 12g, dietary fiber 1g, sugar 6g, protein 5g
Percent Daily Value: vitamin A 45%, vitamin C 89%, iron 6%, calcium 10%

Herbed Romaine with Pine Nuts

preg | can | bones | slim | stress | mood | heart | bloat | skin | time

This salad is simple but elegant and delicious and can be tossed together in under five minutes. The pine nuts add a sophistication and delicious crunch, while the herbs and vinegar are the classy finishing touch. One serving gives you a quarter of your daily fiber quota, a hefty dose of vitamin C, and five times your daily requirement of vitamin A!

Serves 4 (2½ cups per serving)

2 heads romaine, chopped

¼ cup chopped fresh herbs, such as parsley, basil, sage

¼ cup cherry tomatoes

2 tablespoons pine nuts

1 tablespoon extra-virgin olive oil

1 tablespoon balsamic vinegar

1. Wash and chop lettuce into strips, along with fresh herbs. Feel free to use any of your favorite herbs.

2. Halve the cherry tomatoes and throw into salad with pine nuts.

3. Splash olive oil and vinegar on salad and toss until evenly coated.

The pine nuts and olive oil both provide heart-healthy monounsaturated fat and act as a nutrient booster by aiding in the absorption of the fat-soluble beta carotene in the cherry tomatoes.

Per serving: calories 97, total fat 5g, saturated fat 1g, cholesterol 0mg, sodium 28mg, carbohydrates 12g, dietary fiber 7g, sugars 5g, protein 4g
Percent Daily Value: vitamin A 551%, vitamin C 132%, iron 19%, calcium 11%

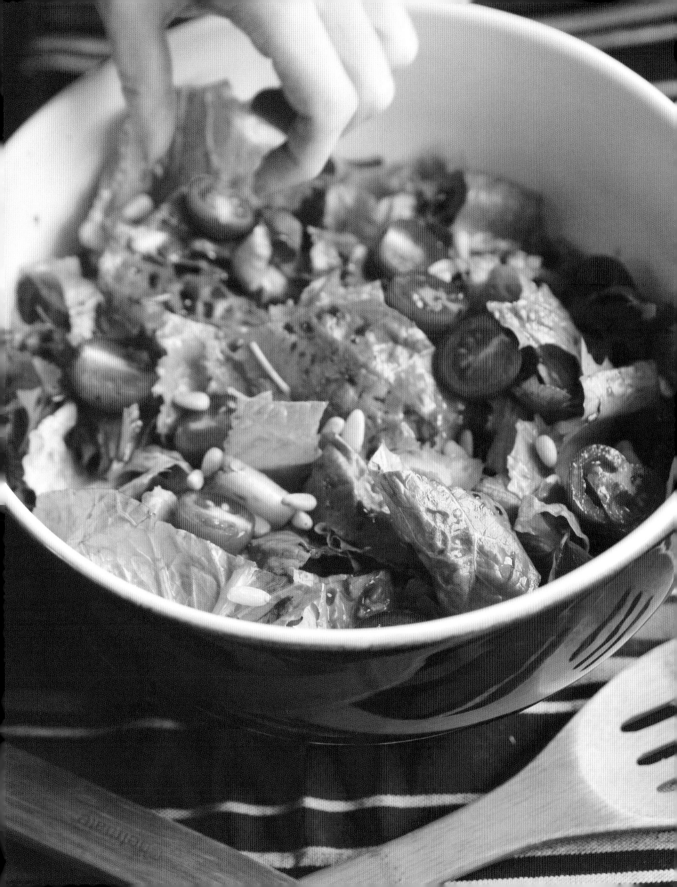

Mojito Salad

can | slim | bloat | skin

Refreshing has found its match! The combination of sweetness, refreshing citrus, and mint flavors is the perfect complement to a backyard barbecue or the ideal starter for a festive meal for a dinner guest. It's no surprise that this salad has a beverage in its name, as it's the ultimate way to hydrate, thanks to its cucumber, which is 96 percent water, and its watermelon, 92 percent. What's more, cucumber and watermelon are the perfect combination to aid in weight loss, since they both fill you up with few calories. So go ahead and "spoil your appetite" with this delicious salad that will help curb your hunger by satisfying your taste buds!

Serves 4 (1¼ cups per serving)

FOR THE SALAD

3 cups watermelon in 1-inch cubes

2 cups peeled cucumber in ½-inch cubes

¼ cup coarsely chopped fresh mint

FOR THE DRESSING

2 tablespoons red wine vinegar

2 tablespoons fresh lime juice

½ teaspoon extra-virgin olive oil

1 teaspoon freshly ground black pepper

2 teaspoons agave nectar or honey

1. Toss together the watermelon, cucumber, and mint. Place in refrigerator and chill for 15 minutes.

2. Mix dressing ingredients with a whisk and pour over salad. Place in refrigerator and chill for 15 minutes more.

3. This refreshing summer salad will pair superbly with grilled fish or will shine at your next summer cookout!

Watermelon not only helps to hydrate your insides with its extremely extraordinary water content, it also hydrates your skin while beautifying it with its high vitamin C and vitamin A content. Watermelon's lycopene will help to keep your skin young by protecting it against sun damage.

Per serving: calories 50, total fat 1g, saturated fat 0g, cholesterol 0g, sodium 5mg, carbohydrates 10g, dietary fiber 1g, sugars 7g, protein 1g
Percent Daily Value: vitamin A 14%, vitamin C 21%, calcium 5%, iron 4%

Ole! Mexican Cabbage with Black Beans and Avocados

heart | can | preg | energy | full | stress | mood | bones | power2 | skin

Although we grew up loving cabbage and thought it was due to our Hungarian ancestry, we'll take this Mexican version any day! We've always been fans of large portions—but we only go for them if the calories are low. Thanks to the low-calorie cabbage, you can get a large serving for few calories. And if you don't want to use avocado, you'll knock off another 65 calories per serving. However, the avocado helps you to absorb more of the skin-beautifying lycopene from the tomato paste. This recipe is simple to prepare but packs a lot of health and flavor. It's quite spicy, so depending on your palate, you may want to reduce the amount of cayenne and jalapeño. This dish is another one whose flavor intensifies when it's refrigerated overnight.

Serves 4 (1 cup per serving)

1. Heat a medium saucepan and add 1 tablespoon of canola oil. Sauté the onion and jalapeño in the pan until they are soft, 3 to 4 minutes.

2. Add the garlic, cumin, oregano, chili powder, pepper, and cayenne and stir into the onion and jalapeño for 1 minute to release the flavor of the spices, then add ¼ cup of water to the pan.

3. Add cabbage, salsa, and tomato paste. When sauce begins to boil, reduce heat and simmer for about 10 minutes or until the cabbage is tender.

4. Remove pan from heat and stir in the cilantro.

5. Add cooked black beans (rinsed well if canned) and avocado slices when ready to serve.

Tip: Use bagged, prewashed, pre-chopped green cabbage. It is a huge time-saver and so convenient!

1 tablespoon canola oil

1 onion, diced

2 jalapeños, diced

2 cloves garlic, minced

1 teaspoon ground cumin

1 teaspoon oregano

1 tablespoon chili powder

¼ teaspoon black pepper

½ teaspoon cayenne pepper

1 pound (about 3⅓ cups) chopped cabbage

¾ cup mild salsa

2 tablespoons low-sodium tomato paste

1 tablespoon chopped cilantro

1 cup cooked no-sodium-added black beans

1 cup sliced avocado (1 avocado)

Per serving: calories 199, total fat 10g, saturated fat 1g, cholesterol 0mg, sodium 287mg, carbohydrates 25g, dietary fiber 9g, sugars 6g, protein 7g
Percent Daily Value: vitamin A 21%, vitamin C 75%, calcium 7%, iron 14%

Red Cabbage Salad with Grapes and Ginger Dressing

slim | heart | can | bloat | skin | stress

We enjoy this salad frequently alongside a nicely grilled piece of fish. The grapes are a pleasant surprise, as they blend in so well with the cabbage. If your grapes are on the large side, you may want to quarter them instead of just halving them. The amount of sugar you should use in this recipe depends on your personal preference. Start with 1 teaspoon and taste the salad; if it's too tart for you, continue adding to taste.

Serves 4 (½ cup per serving)

3 cups shredded red cabbage

1 cup halved seedless red grapes

3 tablespoons fresh lemon juice

1½ tablespoons canola oil

1½ teaspoons sugar, or more to taste

1 teaspoon grated fresh ginger

Salt to taste

Combine all ingredients in a medium bowl.

Grapes are good for your brain! Grapes seem to help protect brain health by counteracting oxidative stress and inflammation, and by fighting age-related diseases of the brain.

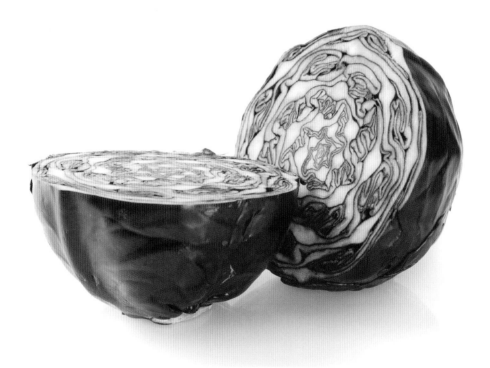

Per serving (without added salt): calories 97, total fat 5g, saturated fat 0g, cholesterol 0mg, sodium 17mg, carbohydrates 13g, dietary fiber 1g, sugars 10g, protein 1g
Percent Daily Value: vitamin A 12%, vitamin C 61%, iron 3%, calcium 3%

Refreshing Beet and Watermelon Detox Salad

heart | can | bloat | skin | stress | mood | detox

This dish is light, refreshing, and delicious with a combination of sweet watermelon, tangy beets, and a hint of citrusy cilantro. It's perfect for a barbecue or a picnic. You get the detox benefits of the beets and the hydration from the watermelon, as well as the skin- and health-protecting benefits of watermelon's vitamin C and lycopene.

Serves 4 (¾ cup per serving)

1. To cook fresh beets, wash, peel, and cut into ½-inch cubes. Place on a foil-lined cookie sheet and bake in a 400°F oven for 45 minutes or until tender.

2. If using canned beets, drain and slice into 1-inch pieces. Place in a bowl with watermelon.

3. Wash and chop cilantro, if using, and add to beets and watermelon.

4. In another bowl whisk together yogurt, balsamic vinegar, lemon juice, olive oil, and salt and pepper.

5. Pour over beets and watermelon and toss until evenly coated.

1 (15-ounce) can sliced beets, no-salt-added preferred, or 1 pound fresh beets or 5 medium (2-inch diameter) beets

1 cup watermelon, in 1-inch cubes

2 tablespoons chopped cilantro (optional)

2 tablespoons fat-free Greek yogurt

2 tablespoons balsamic vinegar

1 teaspoon lemon juice

1 tablespoon extra-virgin olive oil

Salt and pepper to taste

Per serving (with no-salt-added canned beets): calories 84, total fat 4g, saturated fat 0g, cholesterol 0mg, sodium 55mg, carbohydrates 12g, dietary fiber 1g, sugars 10g, protein 2g
Percent Daily Value: vitamin A 5%, vitamin C 13%, calcium 3%, iron 5%

Swiss Chard Salad with Red and Golden Beets and Honey Yogurt Vinaigrette

heart | can | bloat | skin | stress | mood | detox | preg

This recipe was perfect for introducing Tammy's kids to both beets and Swiss chard, toughies for kids. Luckily, the mild, slightly sweet chard went over well, and they loved the salad. The California raisins add a hefty dose of antioxidants and iron and just the right amount of sweet, while the pistachios are packed with fiber and protein and offer a winning combo of crunchy and savory.

Serves 6 (1 cup salad and 1 ounce dressing per serving)

FOR THE SALAD

2 medium yellow beets, scrubbed

2 medium red beets, scrubbed

6 cups Swiss chard, washed and sliced into ½-inch ribbons

½ cup unsweetened California raisins

¼ cup chopped pistachios or cashews, dry-roasted and unsalted

FOR THE HONEY YOGURT VINAIGRETTE

6 ounces (1 small container) nonfat Greek yogurt

1 tablespoon extra-virgin olive oil

2 tablespoons red wine vinegar

Salt and pepper to taste

2 tablespoons honey

1. In a medium-size saucepan, heat enough water to cover the beets. When the water boils, add the whole beets and simmer for 30 minutes.

2. Prepare the vinaigrette while beets are simmering. Whisk together water, yogurt, olive oil, red wine vinegar, and salt and pepper to taste. While still whisking, add the honey.

3. Place the Swiss chard in a large salad bowl.

4. Put raisins in a small bowl and add warm water to cover. Soak for 5 minutes and then drain.

5. Drain the beets and run them under cold water to cool. With a peeler, remove the skin, then slice the beets into ¼-inch cubes or thin half moons.

6. Add the beets to the Swiss chard and garnish with the pistachios and raisins. Drizzle with the vinaigrette.

Per serving (with 2 tablespoons dressing): calories 120, total fat 3.5g, saturated fat 1g, cholesterol 0mg, sodium 122mg, carbohydrates 20g, dietary fiber 3g, sugars 14g, protein 4g
Percent Daily Value: vitamin A 44%, vitamin C 23%, calcium 7%, iron 10%

Veggie Yard Dash Salad

energy | full | time | slim | bloat | skin | heart | can | kid | preg | stress | mood | bones

This zesty salad is the ultimate yummy, not your ordinary salad designed for those on the go. Everything is bagged, jarred, or canned, so all you have to do is toss it all together and it will put an end to the problem of getting your veggie servings!

Serves 4

1. Drain red pepper, black beans, and corn well and place in a large bowl.

2. Add spinach, water chestnuts, artichokes, and sunflower seeds to the same large bowl. Mix well.

3. Drizzle with our Herbed Vinaigrette, or your favorite low-fat vinaigrette, and serve!

¼ cup jarred roasted red pepper, cut into strips

½ cup no-salt-added canned black beans

1 cup no-salt-added canned corn

8 ounces raw baby spinach

1 (4-ounce) can sliced water chestnuts

¼ cup canned sliced artichokes

2 tablespoons raw sunflower seeds

½ cup Herbed Vinaigrette (recipe follows)

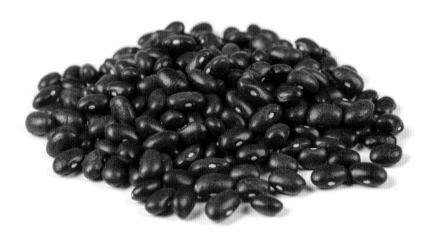

Per serving (not including dressing): calories 134, total fat 3g, saturated fat 20g, cholesterol 0mg, sodium 198mg, carbohydrates 24g, dietary fiber 5g, sugars 2g, protein 6g
Percent Daily Value: vitamin A 107%, vitamin C 43%, calcium 7%, iron 15%

Herbed Vinaigrette

heart | can

This dressing is packed with flavor, not calories and salt. So you can enjoy your salad and all of its health-promoting benefits without having to worry about it bloating you or hurting your waistline. The vinaigrette can be prepared in minutes, and you can keep it in your fridge so that you always have a healthy, tasty dressing on hand.

Serves 4 (1 ounce per serving)

1 garlic clove

2 tablespoons red wine vinegar

1 tablespoon extra-virgin olive oil

¼ teaspoon black pepper

⅛ teaspoon dried oregano

⅛ teaspoon dried basil

⅛ teaspoon salt

1. Crush garlic and let it sit for 5 minutes to release its health-promoting qualities.

2. Combine all ingredients in a bowl and whisk together.

3. Pour over your salad or use as a dip for your favorite vegetables.

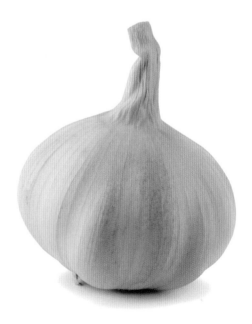

Per serving: calories 29, total fat 3g, saturated fat 0g, cholesterol 0mg, sodium 66mg, carbohydrates 1g, dietary fiber 0g, sugars 0g, protein 0g
Percent Daily Value: vitamin A 1%, vitamin C 1%, iron 1%, calcium 0%

Butternut and Turnip Barley Risotto

heart | can | preg | kid | bones | bloat | skin | energy | full | stress | mood | detox

If you are looking for a delicious and hearty comfort food, you're in luck! Cozy up with this barley risotto, and you'll sink your teeth into a satiating meal that relaxes you while its high-fiber wholesome barley and butternut combo gives you the energy boost you crave. Toasting the barley creates a wonderful, even nuttier flavor, while the orange juice adds a light citrus element that complements the butternut squash. The fresh thyme adds the finishing touch—a fresh herbal bouquet.

Serves 4 (1 cup per serving)

1. **Preheat oven to 350°F. Spread the barley on a cookie pan and toast in the oven for 15 minutes or until the barley is a nutty brown.**

2. **Add the olive oil to a large, heavy-bottomed pot over medium-high heat. Add the leek and sauté for 5 to 7 minutes or until tender.**

3. **Add the toasted barley, thyme, and garlic and cook for 1 minute more, stirring to coat the grain.**

4. **Reduce the heat to medium. Add the orange juice and bay leaf and cook until juice has evaporated, stirring occasionally. Add 1 cup water. Cook, stirring now and then, until the water is absorbed, about 10 minutes. Repeat twice, using 1 cup of water each time, stirring and cooking until the water is mostly absorbed.**

5. **Stir in a fourth cup of water, the butternut squash, turnip, and sage. Cover, reduce heat, and simmer for 20 minutes, stirring every so often. Add the brussels sprout leaves and cook for an additional 15 minutes or until the squash and turnips are tender. Remove from the heat. Stir in the black pepper and Parmesan cheese.**

6. **Serve immediately.**

1 cup uncooked pearl barley

1 teaspoon olive oil

1 medium leek (white and light green parts only), chopped

1 teaspoon chopped fresh thyme

2 garlic cloves, minced

1 cup fresh-squeezed orange juice

1 bay leaf

1 cup peeled, cubed butternut squash

1 small turnip, peeled and cubed (about ⅔ cup)

1 teaspoon chopped fresh sage

½ cup brussels sprout leaves

½ teaspoon freshly ground black pepper

¼ cup Parmesan cheese, for serving

Per serving: calories 287, total fat 4g, saturated fat 1g, cholesterol 6mg, sodium 131mg, carbohydrates 57g, dietary fiber 11g, sugars 9g, protein 10g
Percent Daily Value: vitamin A 88%, vitamin C 83%, iron 14%, calcium 16%

Cauliflower Crusted Mozzarella Pie

heart | preg | can | kid | slim | stress | mood | detox | skin

This pizza is so good that we actually prefer it to the original! Plus, the cauliflower has the added bonus of being much lighter in calories than dough and has fiber and nutrients that will help you kiss deprivation and stress away with this scrumptious pie!

Serves 2

Olive oil cooking spray

1 teaspoon crushed garlic

1¼ cups riced cauliflower (see tip)

½ cup shredded skim mozzarella

½ cup no-salt-added 1% cottage cheese

1 large egg, lightly beaten

1 large egg white, lightly beaten

1 teaspoon dried oregano, Italian seasoning, or basil

2 tablespoons pizza sauce

Toppings of your choice: mushrooms, peppers, squash, eggplant

3 tablespoons shredded skim or part-skim mozzarella, for topping

1. Preheat oven to 450°F. Spray a baking sheet with olive oil.

2. Crush garlic and allow it to sit for 5 minutes to promote its health-boosting benefits.

3. Place riced cauliflower in a medium bowl. Add cheeses, eggs, garlic, and seasoning and mix with a spatula into a coarse pizza dough. Place on the greased baking sheet. Using your hands, form a pie by pressing down until it's uniformly about 1 inch thick.

4. Bake crust in oven for 15 to 20 minutes or until golden brown. After you take it out, top with pizza sauce and toppings of your choice like mushrooms, green pepper, or yellow squash. Sprinkle with the additional 3 tablespoons of mozzarella and bake for another 7 to 10 minutes or until the cheese is melted.

Tip: To rice the cauliflower: Chop a half head of cauliflower into small pieces and microwave for 6 minutes. Let the cauliflower cool for 5 minutes or run it under cold water in a strainer. Rice it either by using a cheese grater or lightly blending in a food processor, keeping its texture coarse.

Per serving (crust only, using skim mozzarella): calories 138, total fat 3g, saturated fat 1g, cholesterol 113mg, sodium 272mg, carbohydrates 6g, dietary fiber 3g, sugars 3g, protein 22g
Percent Daily Value: vitamin A 9%, vitamin C 49%, calcium 22%, iron 6%
Per serving (with pizza sauce and part skim cheese): calories 170, total fat 5g, saturated fat 2g, cholesterol 118mg, sodium 336mg, carbohydrates 8g, dietary fiber 3g, sugars 3g, protein 23g
Percent Daily Value: vitamin A 10%, vitamin C 51%, calcium 29%, iron 6%

Eggplant Parmesan

heart | can | preg | bones | skin | stress | mood | bones | slim | full

This meal is perfect if you feel like you want to splurge without feeling guilty. It's satisfying and delicious and is great if you have dinner guests. We served this to a group of health-minded friends who were thrilled that they had an entire indulgent, rich-tasting meal for just 230 calories!

Serves 2

1. Preheat oven to 375°F.

2. Spread eggplant slices over a paper towel and sprinkle liberally on both sides with kosher salt. Allow to sit for 1 hour. (This will reduce the natural bitter flavors in the eggplant.)

3. Meanwhile, in a medium bowl blend with an immersion blender the plum tomatoes, tomato paste, and garlic.

4. Rinse the eggplant slices to remove the salt, then dry well.

5. In three separate plates, place the flour, the egg, and the panko crumbs mixed with the parsley and thyme.

6. Dredge each eggplant slice in the flour, then the egg, and lastly the panko mixture.

7. Place breaded eggplant on a greased cookie sheet and bake for 30 minutes. Turn oven to broil and broil each side until golden, about 5 minutes per side.

8. Transfer two eggplant slices to a baking dish large enough to leave room between them. Spoon two heaping tablespoons of sauce on top of each slice. Place a half slice of cheese and a basil leaf on top. Sprinkle with Parmesan cheese. Repeat, ending with a basil leaf on top.

9. Place pan in oven and bake for 10 to 15 minutes or until cheese melts.

1 large eggplant, sliced lengthwise into 1-inch-thick slices (you will need 4)

Kosher salt

⅓ cup canned plum tomatoes

2 tablespoons tomato paste

1 clove garlic

¼ cup all-purpose or whole wheat flour

1 egg, lightly beaten

½ cup unseasoned panko breadcrumbs

1 tablespoon chopped fresh parsley

1 teaspoon chopped fresh thyme

8 fresh basil leaves

2 slices low-fat mozzarella, each split in half

2 tablespoons grated Parmesan

Cooking spray

Per serving: calories 230, total fat 10g, saturated fat 4g, cholesterol 75mg, sodium 281mg, carbohydrates 17g, dietary fiber 6g, sugars 5g, protein 14g
Percent Daily Value: vitamin A 15%, vitamin C 22%, iron 15%, calcium 56%

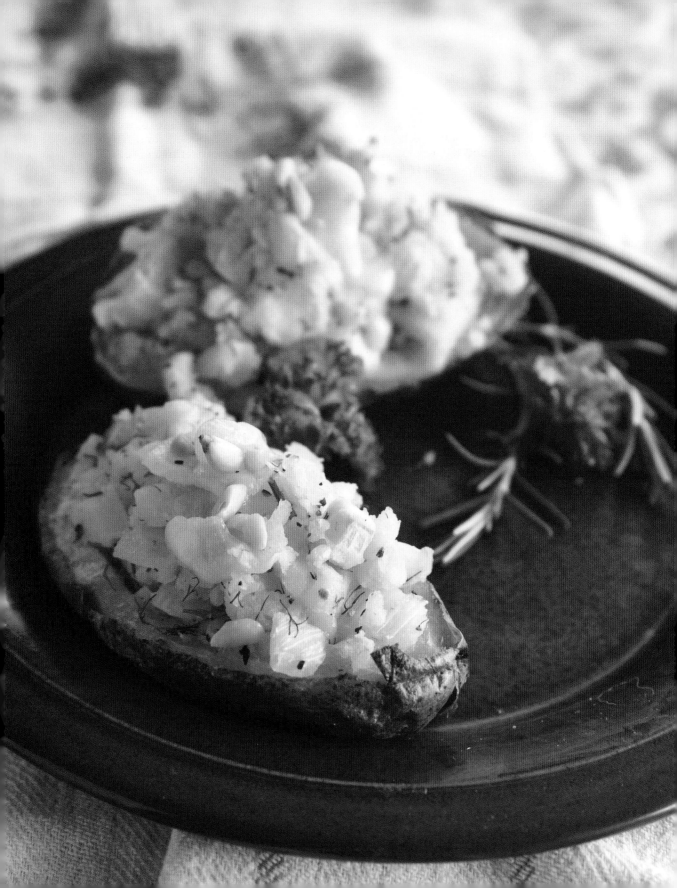

Fennel Stuffed Potatoes

heart | can | slim | preg | bloat | skin | energy | full | stress | mood | detox

When's the last time you had a stuffed *anything* and felt bloat-free? Enter our Fennel Stuffed Potatoes! The combination of the purifying fennel with the potassium-rich potatoes helps to restore fluid balance and will leave you feeling energetic and puff-free. Not bad for a satiating flavor-packed spud! The addition of fennel makes these stuffed potatoes sweet and delish! If you are not fond of the licorice-like flavor of fennel, you can substitute celery for the fennel, dill for the fennel fronds, and then add a bit of dried thyme to compensate for the milder flavor. The Swiss cheese makes it heartier and even more flavorful, and it's hard to believe this entire meal is just over 200 calories.

Serves 4

1. Thoroughly scrub the potatoes and pierce skin in several places with a fork. Bake or microwave until softened (about 40 minutes in a 350°F oven or 8 to 10 minutes in the microwave, turning occasionally). Let cool.

2. While the potato is cooking, in a medium skillet heat the oil on medium-high. Add the fennel, onion, and garlic and cook, stirring, until softened, about 2 minutes. Add the zucchini and cook, stirring, 1 minute longer. Stir in the chopped pignoli and basil. Remove from heat; set aside.

3. When the potatoes are cool, cut in half lengthwise. Scoop out the potato, leaving ¼ inch of flesh in the potato skin. Brush the insides of the potato shells lightly with olive oil and season with salt, if desired; set aside.

4. Measure 1 cup of the scooped potato and place in a medium bowl. Add the broth, fennel fronds, and pepper. Mash until relatively smooth. Stir in the reserved vegetables and all but 2 tablespoons of the cheese. Season with salt, if desired. Spoon the filling mixture into the 4 prepared potato shells. Heat in the oven (350°F for 20 minutes) or microwave (4 minutes on high) until warmed through.

5. Remove from oven and sprinkle tops of potatoes with remaining cheese.

2 large baking potatoes, about 1½ pounds total

1 tablespoon olive oil, plus additional for brushing potatoes

1½ cups fennel in ½-inch dice

½ cup chopped onion

1 clove garlic, minced

½ cup zucchini in ¼-inch dice

2 tablespoons chopped pignoli (pine nuts)

1 tablespoon chopped fresh basil

¼ cup low-sodium vegetable broth or milk

2 teaspoons chopped fennel fronds

¼ teaspoon ground black pepper

⅓ cup shredded low-fat Swiss cheese

Salt to taste

Per serving: calories 217, total fat 7g, saturated fat 1g, cholesterol 2mg, sodium 56mg, carbohydrates 34g, dietary fiber 5g, sugars 2g, protein 7g
Percent Daily Value: vitamin A 3%, vitamin C 36%, calcium 11%, iron 11%

Grab and Go Pita Slaw Sandwich

heart | preg | can | bones | skin | stress | mood | time | slim

This sandwich is a cinch to throw together and perfect after a long day if you don't have much time to cook. It's also an easy way to get your veggies in if you want a quick, healthy lunch. If you're hungry and want something crunchy and satisfying, you've found your match. And if you want an easy sandwich for your kid's lunch box, simply make this and then slice a hard-boiled egg, put it in foil, and let them add it to their sandwich at lunchtime. Prepare this with either our Artichoke Hummus (page 126) or Green Pea Hummus (page 137) instead of a store-bought variety and you'll cut fat and sodium.

Serves 2 (½ large stuffed pita pocket per serving)

1 whole wheat pita

2 cups mixed greens, romaine lettuce, or broccoli slaw

2 teaspoons chopped jalapeño or green bell pepper

4 pieces sun-dried tomato

2 tablespoons hummus, store-bought or ours

1 hard-boiled egg (optional)

1. Cut pita in half and place in toaster if you like it slightly crunchy.

2. Add 1 cup lettuce mix and 1 teaspoon jalapeño or green bell pepper to each pita half.

3. Add sundried tomatoes, hummus, and hard-boiled egg (if desired).

4. Wrap up in foil or a ziplock bag and take on the go!

Tip: We recommend using prewashed and bagged broccoli slaw for this recipe. It looks like shredded carrots, only it's green, and you can find it in the produce section of most stores. It's one of the best inventions to make our lives easier and our food tasty.

Per serving (with broccoli slaw and store-bought hummus): calories 190, total fat 5g, saturated fat 1g, sodium 363mg, carbohydrates 28g, dietary fiber 6g, sugars 4g, protein 11g
Percent Daily Value: vitamin A 15%, vitamin C 138%, calcium 7%, iron 15%

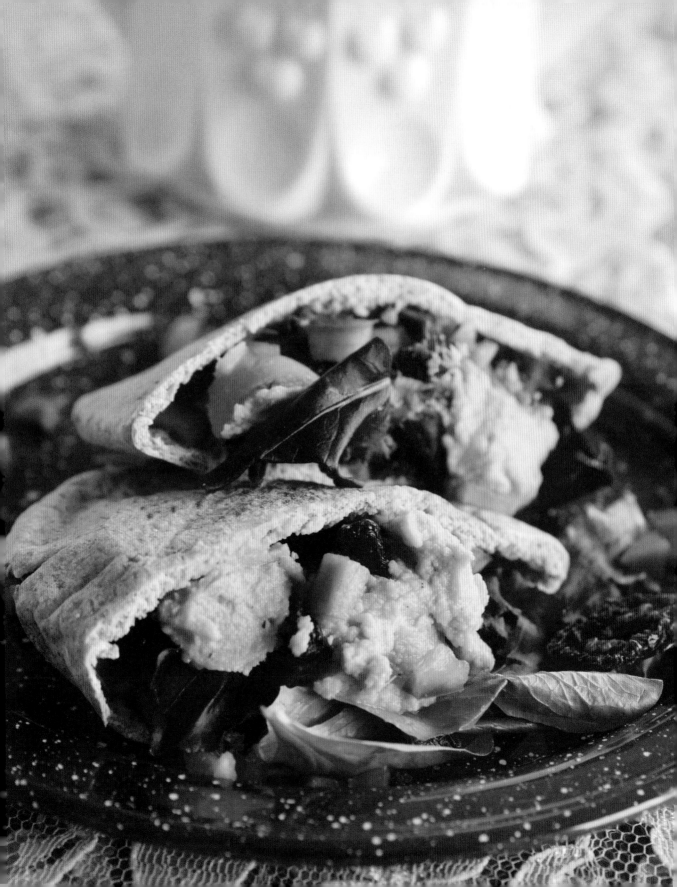

Mediterranean Pizza

heart | can | bones | skin | preg | slim | full | stress | mood

We're big fans of veggie pizzas, and this pizza is the ultimate absolutely scrumptious twist on the original version. The eggplant replaces the standard pizza crust, and it has such a meaty texture that you really feel like you are indulging. This pizza makes a great meal or an afternoon snack for kids. And you get nearly half of your daily recommended fiber when you eat this pizza!

Serves 2

Olive oil cooking spray

2 eggplant slices, cut length-wise, ½ inch thick

¼ cup canned crushed tomatoes, or ½ tomato, cubed and mashed with a fork

½ teaspoon chopped garlic, or 1 garlic clove, pressed

Pinch of Italian seasoning

2 tablespoons shredded part-skim mozzarella

2 tablespoons sliced mushrooms

2 tablespoons chopped green bell pepper

2 tablespoons sliced yellow squash

2 tablespoons chopped onion

2 teaspoons reduced-fat Parmesan-style grated topping

1. Preheat oven to 375°F.

2. Spray a baking sheet with olive oil spray. Pat eggplant slices dry and and place on the baking sheet. Spray slices lightly with olive oil and bake until slightly soft, about 20 minutes.

3. Meanwhile, in a small bowl, prepare the sauce by combining crushed tomatoes, garlic, and Italian seasoning. Mix well and set aside.

4. Take the eggplant out of the oven and evenly spread the tomato sauce over the eggplant slices. Sprinkle with mozzarella and evenly top with mushrooms, pepper, yellow squash, and onion.

5. Bake in the oven until the mozzarella has melted and the toppings are hot, about 10 to 15 additional minutes.

6. Sprinkle with Parmesan and enjoy!

Per serving: calories 193, total fat 4g, saturated fat 1g, cholesterol 5mg, sodium 128mg, carbohydrates 35g, dietary fiber 11g, sugars 20g, protein 11g
Percent Daily Value: vitamin A 110%, vitamin C 157%, calcium 17%, iron 13%

Quinoa with Mixed Vegetables

can | kid | slim | full | skin | detox | heart | preg | stress | mood | bones

If you're looking for a meal that's easy to prepare and that'll get the family to eat more vegetables and whole grains, you've gotta try this. Most people love quinoa, and it's a high-protein, high-fiber healthy alternative to brown rice and whole wheat pasta. The veggies in this dish are mild and an easy way to get your kids to eat their veggies without complaints. The added bonus is that this is easy on the stomach; no one in the family will be constipated after a serving.

Serves 4 (1 cup per serving)

1. On medium heat, pour olive oil in a medium-size pan. Add the onions and sauté for 1 minute. Add the frozen mixed vegetables and simmer for 5 minutes.

2. Add the quinoa to the sautéed vegetables and stir to combine. Add the parsley, lemon juice, lemon zest, and salt and pepper to taste.

3. Garnish with parsley leaves and diced cucumber. Serve.

1 teaspoon olive oil

1 small onion, diced

2 cups frozen mixed vegetables (peas, carrots, corn, green beans)

2 cups cooked quinoa (prepared with water, to package directions)

¼ cup finely chopped parsley, plus a few leaves for garnish

Splash of lemon juice

¼ teaspoon grated lemon zest

Salt and pepper to taste

1 medium seedless cucumber, diced, for garnish

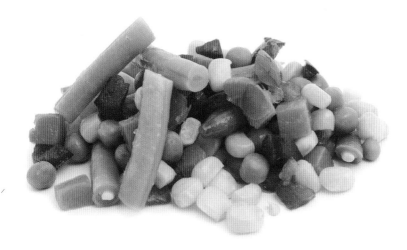

Per serving: calories 207; total fat 4g, saturated fat 1g, cholesterol 0mg, sodium 63mg, carbohydrates 38g, dietary fiber 8g, sugars 2g, protein 8g
Percent Daily Value: vitamin A 121%, vitamin C 34%, iron 16%, calcium 6%

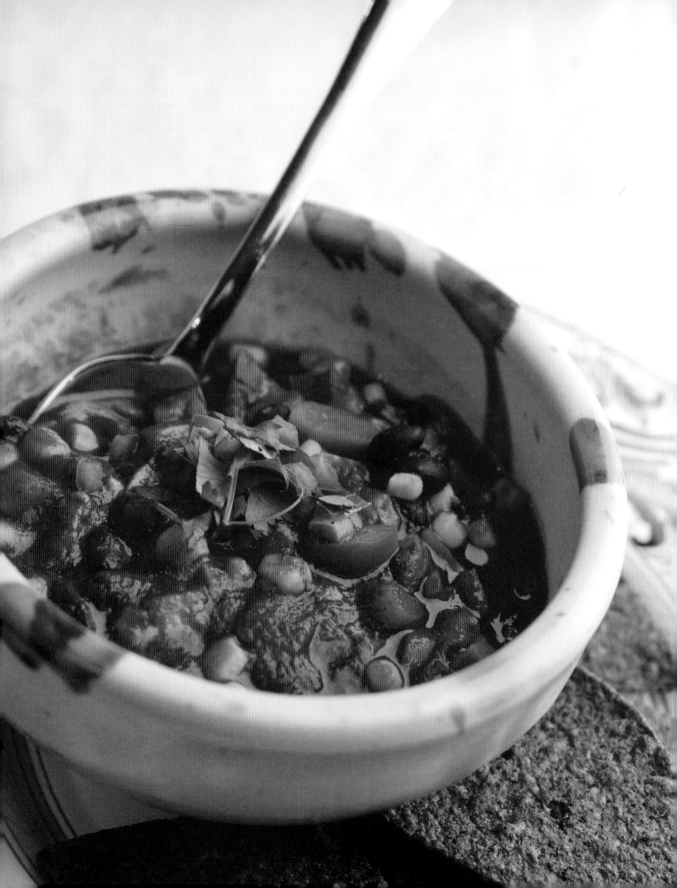

Hot Diggity Chili!

heart | can | preg | energy | full | slim | bones | skin | detox | stress | mood | kid

This hearty chili makes the perfect comfort food. It's delicious and satiating, yet unlike most other comfort foods, it doesn't leave your stomach or your waistline in discomfort. Serve this energy-boosting meal for your Meatless Monday dinner or for Superbowl Sunday, as we do for our families.

Serves 6 (1 cup per serving)

1. In a large pot combine tomato sauce, diced tomatoes, jalapeños, chili powder, and cumin. Stir well and set heat to low.

2. Once sauce starts to boil, add garlic and carrots and cook for 5 minutes.

3. In a skillet "sauté" onions, mushrooms, and peppers in ½ cup water for about 5 minutes or until vegetables soften.

4. Using a slotted spoon, transfer vegetables to pot with sauce, then add corn and beans to chili. Cook over low heat for 2 hours or until carrots are tender. Be sure to stir frequently, about every 20 minutes. You can also use a slow cooker—just leave it and forget about it!

2 (8-ounce) cans no-salt-added tomato sauce

1 cup diced fresh tomatoes

1 tablespoon fresh chopped jalapeño slices

1 teaspoon chili powder

1 teaspoon ground cumin

2 teaspoons crushed garlic

1 cup peeled and chopped carrots

1 cup chopped onions (1–2 onions)

1½ cups chopped portobello mushrooms

1 large red bell pepper, seeded and chopped

1 large green bell pepper, seeded and chopped

1 cup sweet corn kernels, canned or defrosted from frozen, drained

¾ cup canned black beans, drained and rinsed

¾ cup canned red kidney beans, drained and rinsed

Salt to taste (optional)

Per serving: calories 162, total fat 1g, saturated fat 0g, cholesterol 0mg, sodium 118mg, carbohydrates 33g, dietary fiber 8g, sugars 10g, protein 8g
Percent Daily Value: vitamin A 99%, vitamin C 80%, calcium 5%, iron 16%

Roasted Red Pepper, Spinach, and Feta Portobello Burger

power | preg | can | slim | bloat | skin | stress | mood

This burger is to die for! It's bursting with flavor, and if you think you can't sink your teeth into veggies, this portobello burger will prove you wrong. If there is a burger "heaven," you'll feel as if your taste buds are there . . . oh, and so is your happy waistline, since this burger is just 53 delicious calories!

Serves 4

1 red bell pepper

2 cups fresh spinach

4 portobello caps

Olive oil cooking spray

4 tablespoons low-fat or fat-free feta cheese

2 tablespoons balsamic vinegar

Salt and pepper to taste

1. Preheat grill to medium-high.

2. Wash and pat dry the bell pepper, spinach, and portobello caps. Cut pepper into four even pieces.

3. Spray portobello caps and pepper slices with olive oil spray (about 3 sprays per item using a spray bottle, or less than a second spray using a can) to give a light "dusting" of oil.

4. Place on grill, placing the mushrooms with the open side down to start. Grill for about 15 to 20 minutes, flipping the peppers and mushrooms halfway through. When you flip the mushrooms, top with spinach.

5. Once grilled, place one pepper piece on top of each mushroom. Sprinkle with feta cheese and drizzle with balsamic vinegar. Add salt and pepper to taste.

Tip: If you don't have a grill or prefer to stay inside in the colder months, this recipe works just as well broiling the veggies! Broil on high, and the cooking times will be the same.

> Research shows that increasing the intake of lower-calorie foods, specifically mushrooms, in place of those higher in calories, like ground beef, can be an effective method for reducing calories and fat while still feeling full and satisfied after a meal.

Per serving (with fat-free feta and no additional salt): calories 53, total fat 2g, saturated fat 0g, cholesterol 0mg, sodium 25mg, carbohydrates 8g, dietary fiber 2g, sugars 4g, protein 3g
Percent Daily Value: vitamin A 47%, vitamin C 70%, calcium 3%, iron 6%

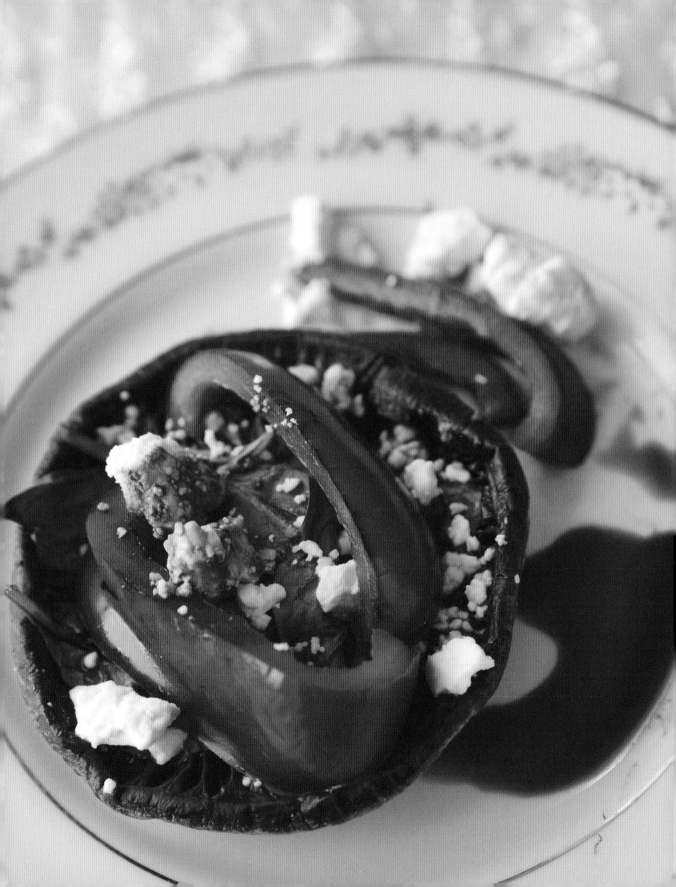

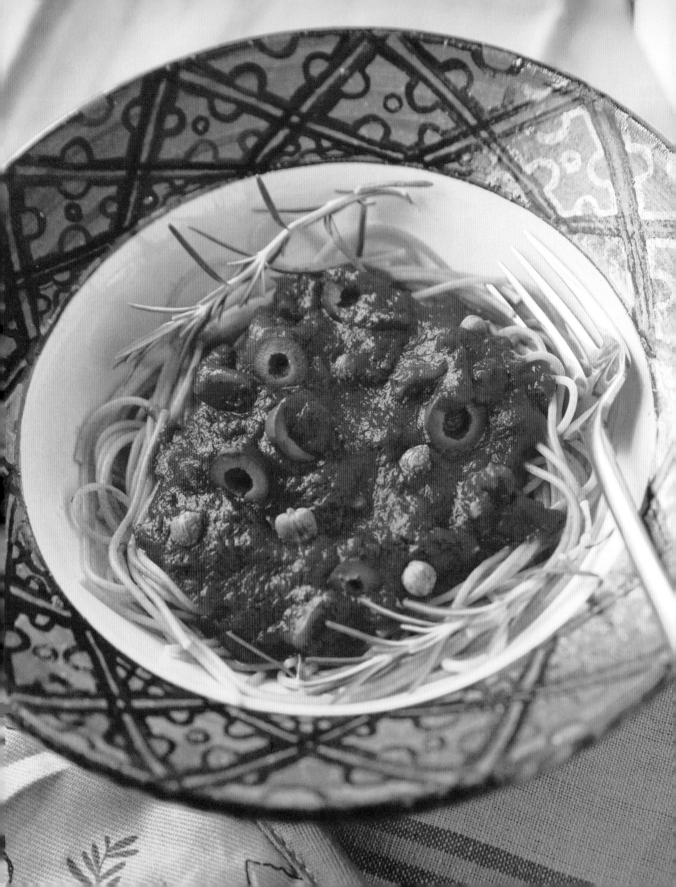

Roasted Tomato Puttanesca

heart | can | preg | bloat | stress | mood | bones | skin

This Puttanesca is so flavorful, you may just want to take a spoon and eat it on its own. Or you can serve it over whole wheat pasta. Either way, you'll feel like you are eating at a fine restaurant in Italy.

Serves 4

1. Preheat oven to 400°F. Line a large baking sheet with parchment paper.

2. In a small bowl place the cherry tomatoes, 1 teaspoon of the olive oil, and 1 teaspoon of the sugar. Toss to coat.

3. Roast the tomato halves until wilted and fragrant, about 20 minutes. Remove from the oven and set aside.

4. In a large pan sauté the shallots in the remaining 1 teaspoon of olive oil until soft and translucent. Add the garlic and heat for 1 minute. Add the olives, capers, oregano, and red pepper flakes and sauté for 4 minutes. Turn off the heat and allow to rest in the pan.

5. Place ¼ cup of the roasted tomatoes in a blender along with the Worcestershire sauce, the remaining 1 teaspoon sugar, and 1 tablespoon water. Puree until smooth. Add the pureed tomatoes to the pan of olives and capers, along with the rest of the roasted tomatoes. Stir gently to combine and heat for 5 minutes or until hot and bubbly.

6. To serve: Toss with ½ pound whole wheat linguine or spaghetti prepared according to package directions.

Note: Allow the cut-up shallots and garlic to sit for at least 5 minutes before cooking to activate the powerful phytonutrient compounds.

Tip: If you'd like extra protein in this meal, try adding cannellini beans, tofu, scallops, or another of your favorite seafoods, or chicken breast.

2 pints cherry tomatoes, sliced in half

2 teaspoons extra-virgin olive oil, divided

2 teaspoons sugar, divided

2 shallots, finely chopped (see note)

2 garlic cloves, thinly sliced

⅓ cup roughly chopped Kalamata olives

2 tablespoons capers, rinsed and roughly chopped

½ tablespoon dried oregano

¼ teaspoon red pepper flakes

1 teaspoon Worcestershire sauce

4 cups cooked whole wheat linguine or spaghetti

Per serving (4 ounces of sauce with 1 cup of pasta): calories 279, total fat 5g, saturated fat 1g, cholesterol 0mg, sodium 262mg, carbohydrates 54g, dietary fiber 9g, sugars 7g, protein 10g
Percent Daily Value: vitamin A 38%, vitamin C 39%, iron 18%, calcium 8%

Spaghetti Squash with Fresh Tomato Sauce

heart | preg | bones | bloat | can | kid | skin | full | energy | stress | mood

This luxurious, rich-tasting meal has all the comfort and satisfaction of pasta but with a fraction of the calories and a lot of extra nutrients from the spaghetti squash and the tomato sauce. The fresh tomato sauce is best made in the summer when tomatoes are ripe and tasty. You can use it on regular pasta or as a sauce for chicken or fish as well, but if you're like us and enjoy great flavor without a lot of calories, opt for the spaghetti squash. Tammy's daughters love to help make this dish by using a fork to dig through and make the "spaghetti."

Serves 2 as main dish (2 cups per serving) or 4 as side dish (1 cup per serving)

1 spaghetti squash (about 3 pounds)

1 tablespoon plus 1 teaspoon extra-virgin olive oil

1 tablespoon minced garlic (3–4 large cloves)

4 cups diced ripe tomatoes

⅓ cup low-sodium tomato or V8 juice

1 teaspoon sugar

Pinch of red pepper flakes

1. Pierce the squash in several places with a fork before cooking. Oven method: Bake at 375°F for 1 hour or until soft; set aside until cool enough to handle. Microwave method: Place on two pieces of paper towel and microwave on high for 10 to 12 minutes, rotating and turning squash three times during cooking, until squash gives slightly when pressed; let stand until cool enough to handle.

2. While the squash is cooking, heat the oil in a 2-quart pot. Add the garlic and cook, stirring, for 30 seconds or until oil and garlic are bubbly. Add the tomatoes with any of their juices and the tomato juice, sugar, and red pepper flakes. Cook, uncovered, stirring and mashing the tomatoes occasionally, for 20 minutes or until sauce is thickened.

3. Cut the squash in half widthwise. Scoop out the seeds and discard. Using a fork, pull out the strands of squash and place in a bowl (you should have 4 cups of spaghetti squash strands). Pour sauce over the squash and toss until combined.

Per serving (1 cup): calories 189, total fat 7g, saturated fat 1g, cholesterol 0mg, sodium 78mg, carbohydrates 33g, dietary fiber 2g, sugars 6g, protein 4g
Percent Daily Value: vitamin A 38%, vitamin C 62%, iron 9%, calcium 10%

Tomato Artichoke Pasta Bake

heart | can | bones

This dish is perfect when you want a true comfort food with a little pizazz. Plus, if we skip a strength-training workout at the gym that day, we feel good that it's helping to strengthen our bones!

Serves 8

1. Preheat oven to 350°F.

2. Heat olive oil in a large sauté pan. Add onion, pepper, salt, and garlic and sauté for 4 minutes. Add artichokes and sauté for an additional 5 minutes. Stir in tomatoes and basil and cook for 2 minutes more. Stir in pasta, combining well.

3. Pour into a large casserole dish.

4. Slice goat cheese with herbs into 8 slices. Arrange slices on top of pasta.

5. Place in oven and bake for 20 minutes.

1 tablespoon extra-virgin olive oil

1 small onion, diced

¼ teaspoon freshly ground black pepper

Salt to taste (optional)

1 clove garlic, minced

1 (12-ounce) bag frozen artichoke hearts

1 (14.5-ounce) can diced fire-roasted tomatoes

¼ cup chopped fresh basil, packed

3 cups cooked whole wheat penne pasta

1 (5-ounce) package goat cheese with herbs

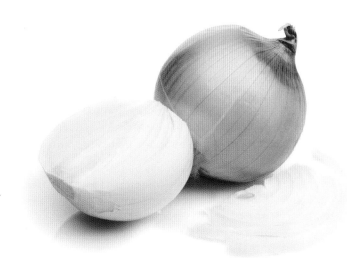

Per serving (without optional salt): calories 172, total fat 7g, saturated fat 4g, cholesterol 14mg, sodium 315mg, carbohydrates 20g, dietary fiber 3g, sugars 1g, protein 8g
Percent Daily Value: vitamin A 11%, vitamin C 10%, iron 7%, calcium 8%

Stuffed Peppers

slim | bloat | skin | full | heart | can | kid | preg | stress | mood

This delicious meal packs in mega-nutrients that will fight cancer, heart disease, and the bloat while giving you a mood boost and fighting wrinkles! But you'll never guess it while your taste buds are rejoicing. When you're preparing it, don't worry if a little of the stuffing falls into the pan when you transfer the peppers from the pan to your serving plate—the stuffing will thicken the sauce nicely. If you find the sauce has turned out too thick for your taste, just add extra broth to it.

Serves 4 (½ pepper per serving)

2 bell peppers (about 8 ounces each), any color

1 tablespoon olive oil, divided

1 cup sliced leek

1½ cups chopped baby portobello mushrooms, divided

¾ cup chopped onion

⅔ cup chopped brussels sprouts

1–1½ cups low-sodium vegetable broth (see page 164), divided

1 tablespoon snipped fresh dill

¼ teaspoon freshly ground black pepper

¾ cup cooked brown rice

¾ cup cooked corn kernels

Salt to taste (optional)

⅓ cup chopped roasted red pepper (see note)

1½ teaspoons balsamic vinegar

Note: Homemade roasted peppers work best. You may use peppers from a jar, but then add ½ teaspoon sugar. You may add more sugar to taste.

1. Preheat oven to 375°F.

2. Cut the peppers in half through the stem. Discard seeds and pith. Cook pepper halves in boiling water for 5 minutes; drain and set aside.

3. In a 10-inch skillet, heat 1½ teaspoons of the oil over medium-high heat. Add the leek and cook, stirring, for 2 minutes or until softened. Add 1 cup of the mushrooms and cook, stirring, for 1 minute longer. Transfer to a 9 x 9-inch baking pan and set aside.

4. Add the remaining 1½ teaspoons of olive oil to the skillet. Add the onion and cook, stirring, for 1 minute; add the brussels sprouts and continue stirring for 1 minute longer. Add the remaining ½ cup mushrooms and cook, stirring, for 1 minute longer or until the vegetables are softened. Stir in ¼ cup of the broth, the dill, and the pepper. Stir in the rice and cook, stirring, for another 1 to 2 minutes or until the broth is absorbed. Add the corn, and salt if desired.

5. Pour ¾ cup of the remaining broth into the pan with the leek mixture. Place the peppers over the leeks in the pan; spoon the rice-corn mixture into the pepper halves. Bake for 20 minutes or until the vegetables in the baking pan are soft and the fillings of the peppers are heated through.

6. Place the peppers on a serving platter or individual serving plates. Pour the broth and vegetables from the pan into a blender or food processor container and add the roasted red pepper and balsamic vinegar. Cover and process until smooth, adding as much of the remaining ½ cup broth as necessary to make a thick but pourable sauce. Serve the sauce with the peppers.

Per serving (using homemade peppers and no salt): calories 179, total fat 6g, saturated fat 1g, cholesterol 0mg, sodium 54mg, carbohydrates 30g, dietary fiber 5g, sugars 7g, protein 5g
Percent Daily Value: vitamin A 25%, vitamin C 210%, calcium 5%, iron 10%

Sweet Potato Veggie Burgers

heart | preg | can | kid | bones | skin | energy | mood | stress

These hearty burgers are a delicious and healthy twist on the traditional burger. You can serve them with lettuce and tomato on a bun. We like the burgers plain (no bun or condiment necessary!), but you can serve them bun-less with tzatziki sauce, a slice of avocado, or guacamole!

Yields 8 burgers

1. In a large bowl, place drained sweet potatoes and beans, and with a fork mash them together until mixed.

2. Add tahini, pepper, and flour and mix again. The mixture will be moist and sticky. Then add the panko crumbs, and with your hands mix them in until you can form patties about the size of your palms. Add more crumbs if the mixture is still too sticky.

3. In a frying pan or skillet, spray canola oil and heat on medium heat. Cook patties on each side for about 2 minutes or until lightly browned.

1 (15.5-ounce) can candied sweet potatoes, or 1¾ cups cooked yams

2 cans low-sodium cannellini beans, rinsed

2 tablespoons tahini

1 teaspoon lemon pepper or cayenne pepper (optional)

¼ cup whole wheat flour

1 cup panko breadcrumbs

Canola oil spray

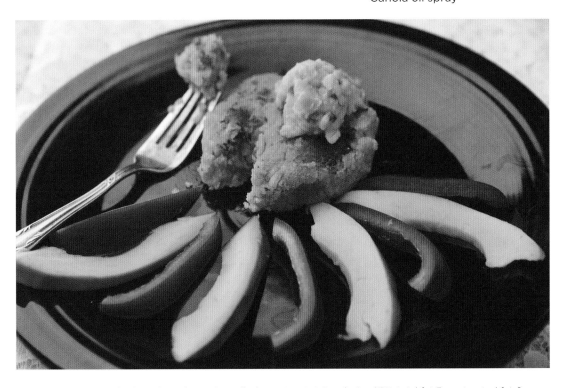

Per serving (with panko breadcrumbs and candied sweet potato): calories 205, total fat 3g, saturated fat 0g, cholesterol 0mg, sodium 25mg, carbohydrates 36g, dietary fiber 6.5g, sugars 5g, protein 9g
Percent Daily Value: vitamin A 6%, vitamin C 2%, calcium 9%, iron 19%

Zucchinilicious Lasagna

heart | can | preg | kid | slim | stress | mood

This lasagna is so fantastic that you'll never want the real deal again. This is the perfect comfort food that'll satisfy your cravings without packing on the pounds. Loaded with fiber and protein but low in calories, you won't believe all of this deliciousness isn't coming from traditional lasagna.

Serves 4 (1 slice per serving)

2½ pounds zucchini, ends trimmed, sliced lengthwise ¼ inch thick

1 teaspoon olive oil

1 cup nonfat ricotta

1 teaspoon garlic powder

1 teaspoon dried oregano

¼ teaspoon freshly ground black pepper

1 cup jarred marinara sauce, Barilla preferred (see note)

¼ cup shredded nonfat mozzarella

Note: You can make this with a low-sodium marinara sauce if you choose to reduce the sodium further. Although we usually recommend doing so, this dish is so delicious as is that we kept the sauce, simply adjusting the other ingredients to help keep the sodium in check.

1. Preheat the oven to 375°F. Line two large baking sheets with parchment paper.

2. In a large bowl toss the zucchini with the olive oil. Arrange the slices in a single layer on the prepared sheets. It's fine if some need to overlap. Roast until soft and flexible like a boiled pasta sheet, about 15 minutes. Set aside.

3. Meanwhile, in a small bowl mix the ricotta with the garlic powder, oregano, and pepper.

4. When the zucchini is cool enough to handle, begin assembly by spreading 3 tablespoons of marinara sauce in the bottom of a 9 x 7-inch oven-safe baking dish. Add a layer of zucchini, slightly overlapping the edges. Spread 2 tablespoons of the seasoned ricotta in a thin layer across the zucchini, then spread 2 tablespoons of marinara evenly across the ricotta. Add another layer of zucchini crosswise to the first. Cut the zucchini to "patch" the layer as needed.

5. Repeat with the ricotta and the sauce until you have five thin layers, ending with a sixth and final layer of plain zucchini on top. Cover the top with the remaining marinara sauce and the mozzarella.

6. Bake uncovered until the top is lightly browned, about 40 minutes. Allow the lasagna to cool for 20 minutes before slicing.

Tip: For perfectly thin and uniform layers, use a mandoline or an Asian-style vegetable slicer.

Per serving (prepared with Barilla marinara): calories 151, total fat 3g, saturated fat 0g, cholesterol 5mg, sodium 387mg, carbohydrates 16g, dietary fiber 4g, sugars 9g, protein 16g
Percent Daily Value: vitamin A 32%, vitamin C 94%, iron 7%, calcium 13%

Bengali Cabbage

slim | heart | can | full | can | skin | stress | mood | detox

This Indian-style dish is easy to prepare, and the flavorful spices are a great contrast to the sweet raisins. The toasted cumin seeds add a warmness that seals the deal. If you save some for another meal, the flavors continue to develop and it gets even more delicious. Although this is a side, the portion is large, as cabbage is low in calories and a great weight-loss food. In fact, you'll find yourself needing fewer heavy foods at the meal. Hello, satisfied and slim!

Serves 4 (1½ cups per serving)

1. In a small bowl add hot water to the raisins to cover. In another small bowl combine the curry powder, turmeric, and cayenne. Add 1 tablespoon water and stir to form a paste. Add ½ cup water and stir until combined, forming the curry sauce. Set aside.

2. In a large pan heat the canola oil over medium heat. Add the jalapeño. Cook for 1 minute. Add the mustard seeds and heat just until the first seed pops, then add the cumin and fennel seeds. Heat for 10 seconds. Add the curry sauce and ginger and give a quick stir. Add the cabbage ribbons and toss. Cover and cook until the cabbage is tender, about 10 minutes, tossing often. Drain the raisins of the soaking liquid and add to the cabbage before serving.

Tip: Have all of your ingredients ready, and read the directions before you fire up the pan. This recipe is super easy but moves quickly between steps.

⅓ cup diced raisins

1 tablespoon curry powder

¼ teaspoon turmeric

¼ teaspoon cayenne pepper

½ tablespoon canola oil

1 teaspoon diced jalapeño

½ teaspoon mustard seed

¼ teaspoon cumin seed

¼ teaspoon fennel seed

¼ tablespoon freshly grated ginger

½ large or 1 small green cabbage (about 2 pounds), cored and sliced into ¼-inch ribbons

Did you know? Although deliciously sweet, California raisins are found to contain compounds that may inhibit growth of the bacteria associated with tooth and gum disease, not contribute to it.

Per serving: calories 114, total fat 4g, saturated fat 0g, cholesterol 0mg, sodium 23mg, carbohydrates 19g, dietary fiber 4g, sugars 12g, protein 2g
Percent Daily Value: vitamin A 7%, vitamin C 73%, iron 9%, calcium 7%

Baby Bellas and Asparagus

heart | can | full | time | preg | bones | kid | bloat | mood | stress

We toss this recipe together when time is tight. We love that it captures the true flavor of both the asparagus and mushrooms and enhances their natural taste. If you aren't watching your weight, feel free to add more oil. Scrumptious in minutes never tasted so good.

Serves 3 (generous ¾ cup per serving)

1 tablespoon extra-virgin olive oil

6 garlic cloves, chopped

2 cups sliced crimini (a.k.a. baby bella) mushrooms (about 8 large mushrooms)

2 cups (about 6 ounces) asparagus spears, cut into 2½–3-inch pieces

Cracked pepper (or substitute ground black pepper) to taste

Sprinkling of red pepper flakes (optional)

1. In a medium-size pan, heat the oil over medium heat. Add garlic and continuing stirring until browned.

2. Add mushrooms and asparagus and stir until asparagus is tender, approximately 3 to 4 minutes.

3. Add black pepper and red pepper flakes (if desired) and serve.

Tip: For perfectly thin and uniform layers, use a mandoline or an Asian-style vegetable slicer.

Tip: Feeling stressed and experiencing the overeating that often is associated with it? This is the perfect dish to bust that feeling. It will curb cravings and stress eating because asparagus is a great source of vitamin C. Get enough vitamin C and you may actually be able to stop the flow of stress hormones—including those that increase body fat! Plus, asparagus has folic acid and other B vitamins that fight anxiety and depression, and it helps provide an overstressed body with energy so that it doesn't crave a cookie for a quick energy boost.

Another bonus? This recipe helps you lose the bloat! Both asparagus and mushrooms are packed with fiber to prevent digestive woes and flush out the colon so you'll be bloat-free.

Per serving: calories 77, total fat 5g, saturated fat 1g, cholesterol 0mg, sodium 6mg, carbohydrates 7g, dietary fiber 2g, sugars 2g, protein 3g
Percent Daily Value: vitamin A 10%, vitamin C 9%, calcium 4%, iron 10%

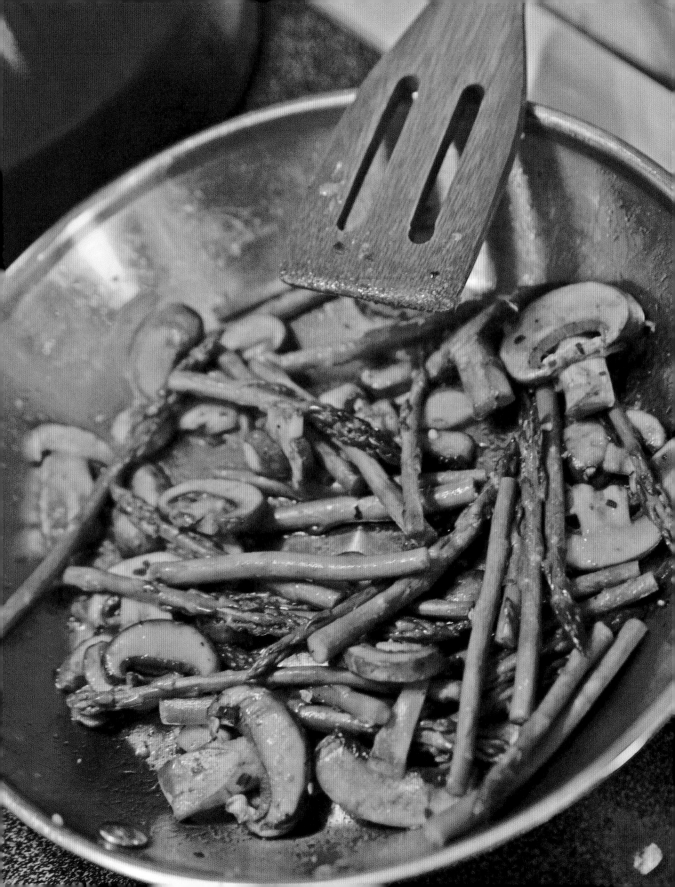

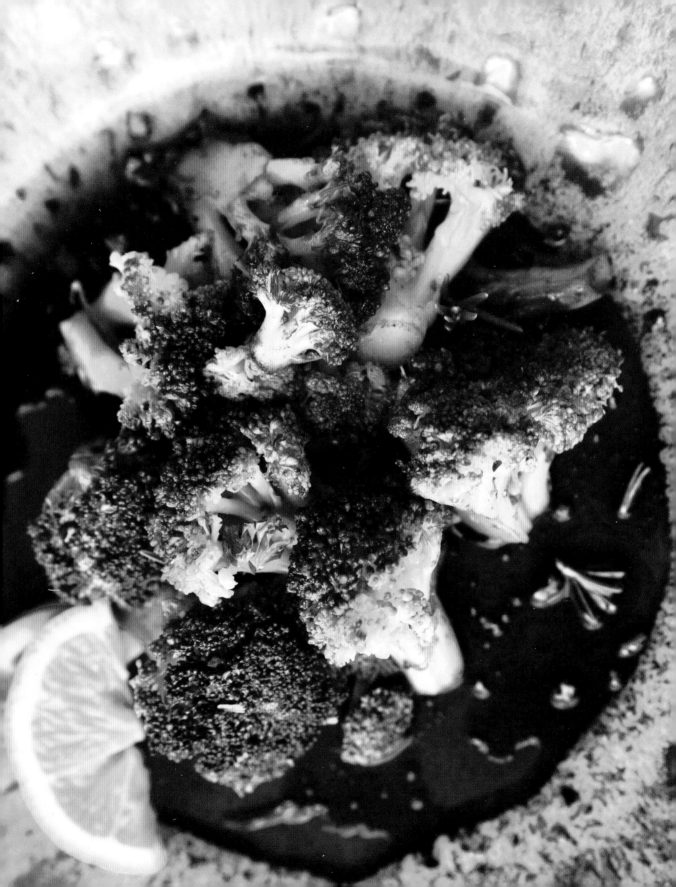

Bangin' Broccoli East Meets West Style

heart | can | kid | skin

This easy Asian-inspired recipe is scrumptious and one of our favorites. We love that it works with nearly any veggie (not just broccoli) and that you can make it any night without having to get fresh produce. This version contains a deliciously (not-so) sweet and sour broccoli with an essence of Provence. It packs in health-promoting fiber. The true beauty is that no one will know that you've used broccoli that's been in your freezer for weeks!

Serves 4 (½ cup per serving)

1. Preheat oven to 400°F.

2. Crush garlic and let it sit for 5 minutes to release all its health-promoting benefits.

3. In a small bowl whisk together all the ingredients except the broccoli.

4. Add the broccoli and toss it in the marinade to coat evenly.

5. Cut a sheet of aluminum foil 12 x 18 inches and fold up the sides like a bowl. Add the marinated broccoli and any liquid left over onto the aluminum foil "pan."

6. Place foil "pan" on a cookie sheet and place in oven.

7. Bake for 20 minutes uncovered or until vegetables are thoroughly cooked through.

8. Enjoy! You can leave it in the foil and wrap the foil into a pouch to take with you on the go!

Note: Herbes de Provence is a mix that may contain any or all of rosemary, thyme, marjoram, basil, bay leaf, summer savory, fennel, chervil, tarragon, and, most distinctively, lavender.

2 cloves garlic

2 tablespoons balsamic vinegar

2 teaspoons low-sodium soy sauce

2 teaspoons packed brown sugar

1 teaspoon olive oil

2 teaspoons herbs de Provence (see note), or oregano or Italian seasoning

½ teaspoon fresh-grated lemon zest

½ teaspoon freshly ground black pepper

2½ cups frozen broccoli

Per serving: calories 56, total fat 1g, saturated fat 0g, sodium 117mg, cholesterol 0g, carbohydrates 9g, dietary fiber 3g, sugars 5g, protein 3g
Percent Daily Value: vitamin A 23%, vitamin C 92%, calcium 7%, iron 6%

Butternut Squash and Mango Mash

heart | can | preg | kid | bones | bloat | skin | energy | full | stress | mood

Lots of taste surprises in this dish. If you can't find morello cherries (sour or tart cherries), you can use dried sour cherries or just canned bing cherries. If the tart flavor and health aspects (see side-bar) appeal to you and you can't find them canned, frozen, or dried, you can buy a can of cherry pie filling and rinse off the goo. We often eat this mash for dessert, and it always hits the spot for us after any meal. And it's a great way to get a burst of energy.

Serves 6 (½ cup per serving)

3 cups peeled butternut squash in 1-inch cubes

1 tablespoon orange juice

1 cup cubed mango

1 cup diced mango

½ cup canned pitted morello (sour) cherries, drained and halved or coarsely chopped

¼ cup finely chopped pecans (optional)

2 tablespoons chopped cilantro

⅛ teaspoon red pepper flakes

¼ teaspoon kosher salt (optional)

1. Place the squash and orange juice into a microwave-safe bowl; microwave on high for 6 minutes, stirring every 2 minutes, or until squash is soft. Put the squash with any liquid from cooking into a food processor container fitted with a steel blade. Add the cubed mango, cover, and process until pureed.

2. Return the puree to the microwave-safe bowl. Stir in the diced mango, cherries, pecans (if using), cilantro, pepper flakes, and salt (if using).

3. Microwave on high for 1 to 2 minutes or until heated through.

> The sweet-tart taste of tart cherries adds another dimension to this recipe. It's distinctive enough to stand out, but also subtle enough to complement other flavors. Packed with powerful antioxidants that offer anti-inflammatory benefits, and also a good source of potassium, tart cherries help to relax your body. Added bonus? Tart cherries are linked to reduced pain from gout and arthritis and have an extensive list of heart-healthy benefits. Recent studies even suggest tart cherries can help reduce post-exercise muscle and joint pain.

Per serving (without addition of salt): calories 162, total fat 5g, saturated fat 1g, cholesterol 0mg, sodium 57mg, carbohydrates 31g, dietary fiber 5g, sugars 17g, protein 3g
Percent Daily Value: vitamin A 251%, vitamin C 82%, iron 9%, calcium 7%

Cool Cucumber Bites

can | slim | bloat | skin

These crisp and refreshing nibbles make fabulous "grab-it" snacks. They're simple to make and the perfect crunchy way to take the edge off of hunger while helping you to feel light and lean. The freshly ground pepper adds a great zest, so you may not even find it necessary to add salt. You can adjust the amount of seasonings you use to match your own preferences.

Serves 1 (about 1½ cups sliced)

1. Peel the cucumbers and cut them into coin-shaped slices. Place cucumber rounds on a plate and spray with olive oil so that the entire surface of the cucumber gets spritzed, about ½ teaspoon's worth.

2. Sprinkle lemon juice over the slices. Grind pepper over them and add a dash of chili powder. Salt to taste.

Tip: If baby cucumbers are not available, you can use a cucumber of the regular variety. After you peel it, simply cut it in half lengthwise before slicing it into half rounds.

1–2 baby cucumbers

Olive oil cooking spray

1 teaspoon lemon juice

Dash of freshly ground pepper, or to taste

Dash of chili powder, or to taste

Salt to taste (optional)

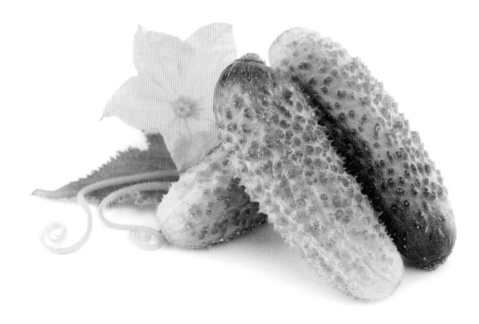

Per serving: 37 calories, total fat 2g, saturated fat 0g, cholesterol 0g, sodium 4mg, carbohydrates 3g, dietary fiber 1g, sugars 2g, protein 1g
Percent Daily Value: vitamin A 2%, vitamin C 9%, calcium 2%, iron 2%

Chipotle Smashed Sweet Potatoes

heart | preg | can | kid | bones | skin | energy | mood | stress

This sweet and spicy mash is one of our favorites. It's so delicious that it's addictive, and if you're craving energy, kiss your coffee and other caffeine good-bye, this is your new perk.

Serves 4 (½ cup per serving)

4 medium sweet potatoes

½ dried chipotle pepper, stemmed and seeded

2 tablespoons I Can't Believe It's Not Butter! Light

Salt to taste

1. Preheat oven to 400°F.

2. Roast the sweet potatoes in the oven for 45 to 60 minutes or until very soft.

3. Meanwhile, in a coffee grinder or blender, blitz the chipotle pepper until it is finely ground.

4. Carefully remove the skins from the hot potatoes. Place the sweet potatoes in a heatproof bowl and smash them with a fork. Add the I Can't Believe It's Not Butter! and chipotle powder. Mash or blend until smooth and creamy. Salt to taste and serve.

Tip: Can't find dried chipotle peppers? Substitute 1 teaspoon of a chipotle hot sauce like Tabasco or Cholula brand for the dried pepper.

Per serving (without salt): calories 137, total fat 3g, saturated fat 1g, cholesterol 0mg, sodium 125mg, carbohydrates 27g, dietary fiber 3g, sugars 5g, protein 2g
Percent Daily Value: vitamin A 376%, vitamin C 5%, iron 5%, calcium 4%

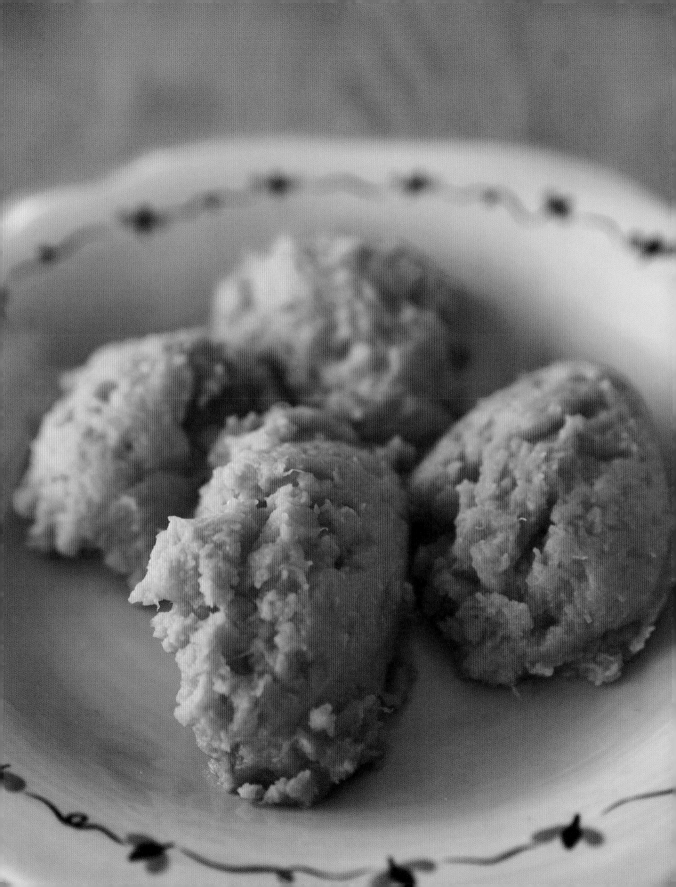

Easy Spinach Pomodoro

heart | can | preg | bones | slim | bloat | skin | full | stress | mood | time

We originally made this dish as a lightened-up lasagna inspired by our mom's vegetarian lasagna. When we realized how much we loved the flavor of the spinach, tomato sauce, and Parmesan and that it was such a quick and easy way to sneak in our nutrients, it became a staple when we were in college. We always felt we could really sink our teeth into it and feel satisfied with just a few calories. Plus, we loved what the spinach and tomatoes did for our skin!

Serves 2

1 (10-ounce) package frozen spinach, or 1 (9–10-ounce) bag raw spinach

¾ cup tomato sauce

2 tablespoons nonfat mozzarella

2 teaspoons grated Parmesan cheese

1. In a medium-size saucepan, prepare the spinach according to package directions. Stir the tomato sauce into the spinach.

2. Add mozzarella to the mixture and stir until cheese melts.

3. Divide spinach into two portions and sprinkle with Parmesan.

Tip: If you have a favorite low-sodium tomato sauce, it will really help to keep the sodium down.

Tip: When choosing a jarred sauce, look for a calorie count of 90 or less per ½-cup serving.

Per serving: calories 86, total fat 2.4g, saturated fat 0.9g, cholesterol 5.1mg, sodium 168mg, carbohydrates 14g, dietary fiber 4.6g, sugars 2g, protein 6g
Percent Daily Value: vitamin A 281%, vitamin C 37%, calcium 23%, iron 15%

Floating Asparagus Rafts

heart | can | preg | bones | kid | bloat | mood | stress

This recipe is perfect when you want a crowd-pleaser for the entire family. Kids love it as much as adults. In our family, we always go around the table and share where we are imagining we would float on our "raft." It always puts us in a good mood—well, the conversation as well as the nutrients in the asparagus.

Serves 4

1. Preheat oven to broil and spray a cookie sheet with cooking spray.

2. Prepare asparagus by removing the tough ends, which will easily snap off. Place asparagus in groups of 4 on the cookie sheet, and thread with 2 toothpicks horizontally through each group.

3. In a small bowl combine soy sauce, sesame oil, and garlic.

4. Brush sauce over asparagus and broil for 4 minutes on each side or until lightly golden.

5. Sprinkle with pepper.

16 asparagus spears (about 1 pound)

½ tablespoon low-sodium soy sauce

1 teaspoon dark sesame oil

1 garlic clove, minced

¼ teaspoon freshly ground black pepper

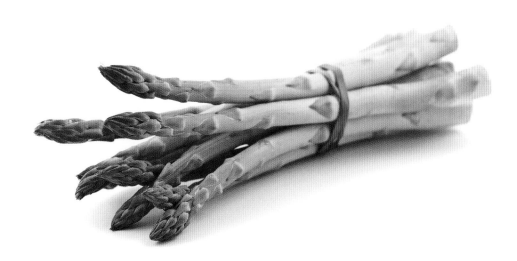

Per serving: calories 22, total fat 1g, saturated fat 0g, cholesterol 0mg, sodium 68mg, carbohydrates 2g, dietary fiber 1g, sugars 1g, protein 1g
Percent Daily Value: vitamin A 7%, vitamin C 5%, iron 6%, calcium 1%

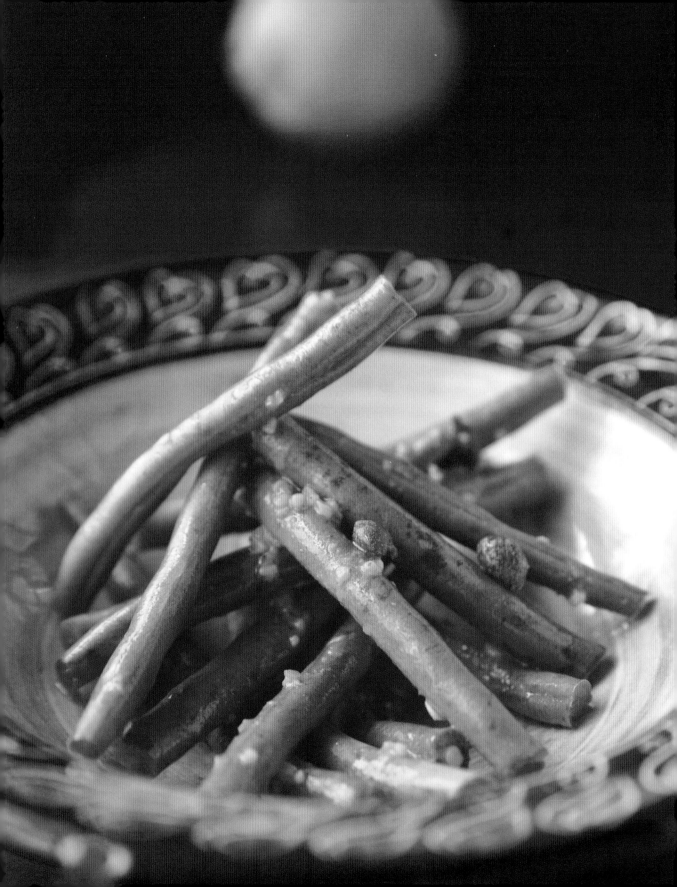

Green Beans with Lemon Caper Vinaigrette

heart | preg | can | bones | kid | stress | mood

This is a great recipe to keep in your back pocket for those nights when you want a veggie with a little pizzazz in a jiffy. We love that there's a lot of flavor and yet the calories stay low due to the minimal amount of oil and the shaved Romano.

Serves 2 (4 ounces per serving)

1. Using a steamer basket inserted into a large saucepan, steam the green beans to desired degree of tenderness, about 5 minutes. They should be bright green and al dente.

2. In a small jar with a tight-fitting lid, place all the ingredients for the vinaigrette. Close the lid tightly and shake until the dressing is well mixed and creamy.

3. Once the beans have cooked, transfer them to a serving bowl. Toss with the vinaigrette and let stand for 10 minutes.

4. Using a grater or microplane, shave about 1 teaspoon of Romano cheese over the green beans before serving. If you only have a peeler, peel small bits of the cheese on top of the green beans.

Note: A microplane helps with both enjoyment and portion control of flavorful foods like Parmesan cheese and chocolate.

½ pound fresh green beans, trimmed

Romano cheese for shaving

FOR THE LEMON CAPER VINAIGRETTE

1½ teaspoons extra-virgin olive oil

½ clove garlic, crushed with a knife

½ teaspoon capers, rinsed and coarsely chopped

Pinch of freshly ground black pepper

½ teaspoon fresh lemon juice

¼ teaspoon Dijon mustard

Per serving: calories 67, total fat 4g, saturated fat 0g, cholesterol 0mg, sodium 39mg, carbohydrates 8g, dietary fiber 4g, sugars 2g, protein 2g
Percent Daily Value: vitamin A 16%, vitamin C 32%, iron 7%, calcium 4%

SIDES

Green Bean Salad with Toasted Almonds and Dates

heart | preg | can | bones | kid | stress | mood

This warm and delightfully sweet and crunchy dish hits the spot. And the dates offer more than just a sweet treat: They are a good source of fiber and higher by weight in polyphenol antioxidants than blueberries. The almonds add a delicate flavor and delectable crunch while providing a boost of phenolics, flavonoids, vitamin E, and other nutrients. We've been known to eat all of the dish before it makes it to the table.

Serves 4 (about ⅔ cup per serving)

1 pound green beans, topped and tailed

½ teaspoon minced garlic

2 tablespoons slivered almonds

¼ cup pitted and chopped dates

Freshly ground black pepper to taste

Pinch of salt (optional)

1. Preheat the oven or toaster oven to 350°F.

2. Steam green beans and garlic together. Meanwhile, toast almonds by spreading them evenly in a baking dish and baking for 2 to 7 minutes, flipping/stirring every minute or two to prevent them from burning.

3. When green beans are crisp-tender, remove from heat and transfer to a large bowl. Add almonds and dates, sprinkle with pepper and salt (if desired), and mix well. Serve while warm.

> **Dates are higher in polyphenol antioxidants than blueberries by weight. They're also a good source of fiber and a delicious and healthy way to sweeten culinary dishes; since dates produce their pure sweet flavor naturally, no added sugar is required.**

Per serving: calories 81, total fat 2g, saturated fat 0g, cholesterol 0g, sodium 42mg, carbohydrates 16g, dietary fiber 5g, sugars 8g, protein 3g
Percent Daily Value: vitamin A 15%, vitamin C 31%, calcium 6%, iron 8%

Heavenly Roasted Vegetables

preg | can | kid | slim | stress | mood | bones | heart | skin | bloat

Yes, just a bite of these and you'll think you went to heaven! These to-die-for veggies are so easy to make that they'll automatically put you in a good mood. Your taste buds will smile, and that's even before all of the mood-boosting vitamin D from the mushrooms makes its way into your body and spirit.

Serves 4 (1 cup per serving)

1. Preheat the oven to 350°F. Line two large baking sheets with parchment paper.

2. Remove seeds from bell peppers and slice into 1-inch strips. Cut squash lengthwise into ½-inch-thick slices and cut slices into 3-inch lengths. Cut mushrooms in half unless they are quite small. Trim asparagus and cut into 3-inch lengths.

3. In a large bowl toss the vegetables with 1 tablespoon olive oil. Spread them out on the two baking sheets and roast for 30 minutes.

4. Meanwhile, whisk the remaining 1 teaspoon of oil, balsamic vinegar, garlic, parsley, basil, rosemary, and black pepper in a small bowl.

5. Drizzle the dressing over the roasted vegetables and toss. Serve the vegetables warm or at room temperature.

2 red bell peppers

2 yellow squash

8 ounces whole white button mushrooms

1 bunch asparagus

1 tablespoon plus 1 teaspoon extra-virgin olive oil

2 tablespoons balsamic vinegar

1 garlic clove, minced

1 teaspoon chopped fresh Italian parsley

1 teaspoon chopped fresh basil leaves

½ teaspoon finely chopped fresh rosemary leaves

¼ teaspoon freshly ground black pepper

> Did you know that mushrooms are nature's hidden treasure for vitamin D, the "sunlight" vitamin? Mushrooms are the only fruit or vegetable that naturally contain vitamin D, a nutrient that many people lack. Higher intake of vitamin D may lower risks for some cancers, including prostate, breast, lung, colon, and colorectal.

Per serving: calories 104, total fat 5g, saturated fat 1g, cholesterol 0mg, sodium 18mg, carbohydrates 13g, dietary fiber 4g, sugars 7g, protein 5g
Percent Daily Value: vitamin A 50%, vitamin C 162%, iron 12%, calcium 4%

Herb and Garlic Creamed Spinach

heart | can | preg | bones | slim | skin | full | stress | mood | time

This mouthwatering dish is so easy that you can make it when you have only a couple of minutes to spare. The spinach will give you a good fiber boost, while the cheese will provide you with a dose of calcium.

Serves 4 (½ cup per serving)

2 cups frozen spinach (10-ounce bag or box), or 1½ pounds fresh spinach

2 wedges Laughing Cow Light Garlic & Herb (or Swiss) cheese

1. If using frozen spinach, heat for about 1 minute in the microwave, draining as much excess water as possible. In a medium-size frying pan, heat frozen spinach or fresh spinach and 2 wedges of cheese.

2. Mix in the cheese with a spatula until spinach is evenly coated and the cheese melts.

3. Heat until spinach is completely wilted, about 2 minutes, and serve as a delicious side dish.

We like Laughing Cow Light cheese wedges as a fabulous way to add great taste to veggies without adding a lot of calories. Each individually wrapped, portioned wedge is 35 calories, and tossing them into veggies makes for a quick and healthy snack or side!

Per serving (with frozen spinach): calories 32, total fat 1g, saturated fat 0g; 1 mg cholesterol, sodium 155mg, dietary fiber 2g, carbohydrates 3g, sugars 1g, protein 3g
Percent Daily Value: vitamin A 185%, vitamin C 15%, calcium 18%, iron 16%

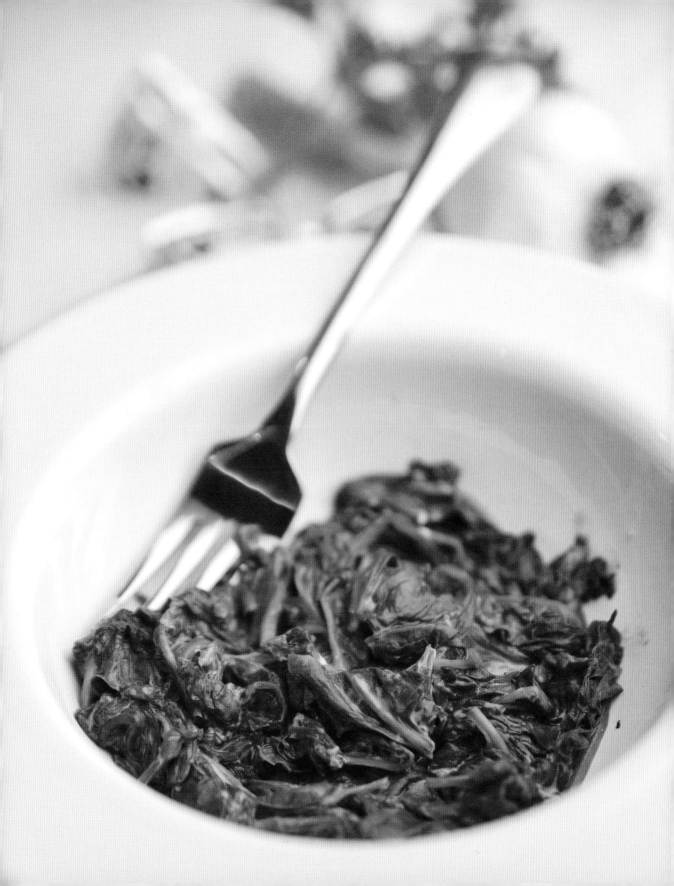

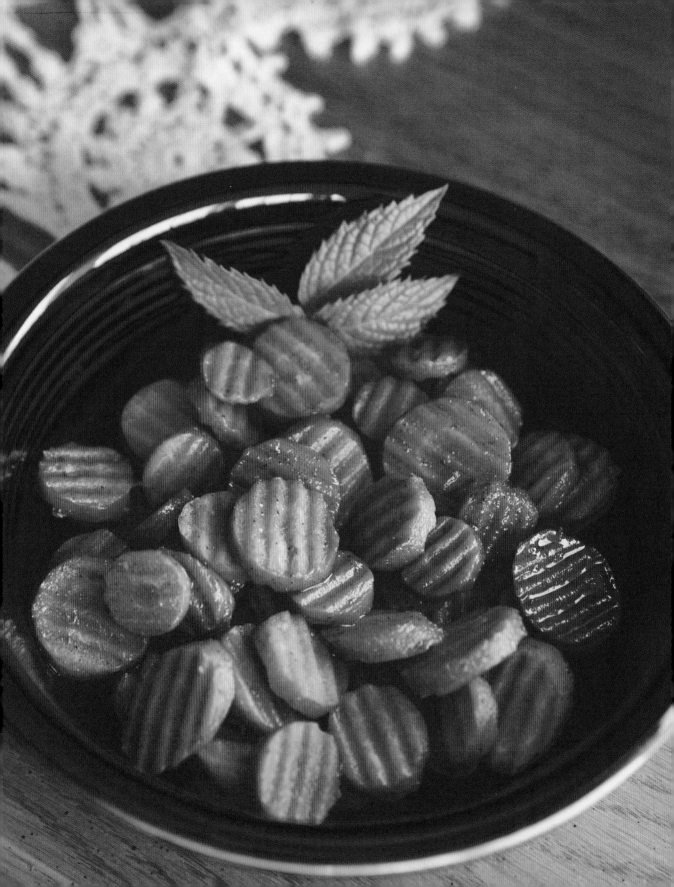

Honey Ginger Carrot Coins

heart | can | kid | slim | full | skin | detox | time

This recipe is so easy and a kid favorite. Tammy's daughters love helping to prepare this dish and take every opportunity to lick the honey as they make it. Best of all, they always ask for seconds, so it helps them to pack in the nutrients. An added bonus? The carrots become even better for you as they cook, as their beta-carotene becomes more absorbable.

Serves 2

1 tablespoon honey

Sprinkling of ground ginger

1⅓ cup carrots (about 4 medium), cut into coins

1. In a medium-size pan, heat honey over low heat. As the honey starts to soften, tilt the pan so honey covers the bottom.

2. Lightly sprinkle ginger powder over entire surface area of honey.

3. Add carrots and cook over medium-high heat until carrots become slightly tender, about 4 minutes—longer if you prefer softer carrots—and serve.

Anyone in the family feel a cough coming on? Try having this for dinner. Honey seems to be a natural cough suppressant! Just a small dose of honey given before bedtime provided the greatest improvement of nighttime cough and sleep difficulty in children over one year of age when compared to dextromethorphan and to no treatment.

Per serving: calories 65, total fat 0g, saturated fat 0g, cholesterol 0mg, sodium 42mg, carbohydrates 16g, dietary fiber 2g, sugars 12g, protein 1g
Percent Daily Value: vitamin A 271%, vitamin C 8%, calcium 3%, iron 2%

Italian Mushrooms, Tomato, and Spinach

heart | can | full | stress | mood | bones | power2 | slim | bloat | skin

This dish has a subtle warmth from the wine and a really rich flavor despite being low in fat. We especially enjoy it on a cold day. It's packed with nutrients, and the vitamin C in the tomato helps the iron from the spinach to be absorbed, giving a real nutrition punch.

Serves 4 (½ cup per serving)

1 tablespoon extra-virgin olive oil

1 small onion, chopped

2 cloves garlic, chopped

1 large tomato, cubed

14 ounces portobello mushrooms, sliced

10 ounces spinach, roughly chopped

1 tablespoon balsamic vinegar

¼ cup dry white wine

Salt and freshly ground black pepper to taste

Parsley for garnish (optional)

1. In a large skillet, heat the olive oil on medium-high heat. Sauté onion and garlic in the oil until they start to become lightly brown and opaque, about 3 to 4 minutes. Add the tomatoes and mushrooms. Once the tomatoes and garlic start to shrink, toss in spinach. Stir until spinach is wilted.

2. Continue stirring and add the vinegar.

3. Once the vinegar is absorbed, stir in the white wine.

4. Simmer the mixture on low until wine is almost completely absorbed, about 20 minutes. Season with salt and pepper to taste, and garnish with fresh parsley (if desired). Serve hot as a side or on top of your favorite meat or fish.

Per serving: calories 96, total fat 4g, saturated fat 1g, cholesterol 0mg, sodium 64mg, carbohydrates 11g, dietary fiber 3g, sugars 4g, protein 5g
Percent Daily Value: vitamin A 131%, vitamin C 36%, calcium 9%, iron 15%

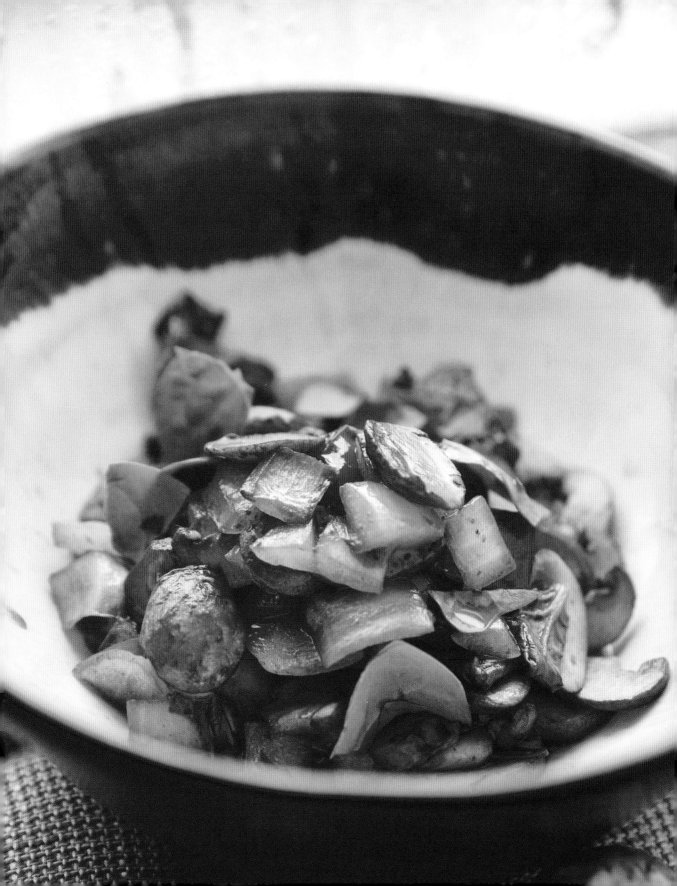

Jicama Fried Rice

heart | can

This "fried rice" doesn't contain any rice at all, just jicama chopped to look like rice. The resulting dish is a little crunchy, slightly sweet, and extremely delicious. Your digestive tract will love you for the fiber, and your heart will thank you for the nutrients that keep it healthy too. We can't get enough of it!

Serves 4 (generous ½ cup per serving)

2 cups peeled, cubed jicama

¼ cup low-sodium vegetable broth

1 tablespoon mirin or dry sherry

2 teaspoons low-sodium soy sauce

1 teaspoon sugar

1 tablespoon vegetable oil

2 teaspoons minced ginger

1 large clove garlic, minced

½ cup chopped carrots

½ cup chopped snow peas

½ cup lightly packed chopped watercress or bok choy

⅓ cup sliced scallion

1. Place the jicama in a food processor fitted with a steel blade. Process on pulse until the jicama is the size of grains of rice; set aside.

2. In a small bowl stir together the broth, mirin or sherry, soy sauce, and sugar.

3. In a large skillet heat the oil over high heat. Add the ginger and garlic and cook, stirring, for 30 seconds. Add the carrots and snow peas. Cook, stirring, for 2 minutes. Add the jicama, watercress or bok choy, and scallion and cook, stirring, for 2 minutes longer. Add the broth mixture. Cook, stirring, for about 3 minutes or until all the liquid has evaporated.

Per serving: calories 90, total fat 4g, saturated fat 0g, cholesterol 0mg, sodium 114mg, carbohydrates 10g, dietary fiber 4g, sugars 3g, protein 1g
Percent Daily Value: vitamin A 61%, vitamin C 40%, calcium 3%, iron 5%

Kung Pao Veggies

can | kid | slim | full | skin | detox

This dish was inspired by the fiery chicken dish that gives your taste buds a kick and really wakes up your senses—and your entire body. This dish will do the same, but without all of the artery-clogging calories from the fried original version.

Serves 4

1. Let the sliced scallions sit for 5 minutes to allow their health-promoting antioxidants to develop.

2. Seed the chile peppers and break them into small pieces.

3. In a small bowl mix together soy sauce, rice vinegar, sugar, cornstarch, and 3 tablespoons water.

4. In a large skillet or wok, heat the oil. Add the scallions and chile peppers, and stir-fry for 1 minute. Add the bok choy, ginger, carrot, and peanuts (if using) and stir-fry for 1 minute more. Pour the sauce over the mixture and stir until it thickens and bubbles.

½ cup sliced scallions

2 dried red chile peppers

1 tablespoon reduced-sodium soy sauce

2 tablespoons rice vinegar

½ tablespoon granulated sugar

1 teaspoon cornstarch

2 teaspoons canola oil

2 cups coarsely chopped bok choy

1 teaspoon grated fresh ginger, or ¼ teaspoon powdered ginger

1 cup grated carrot

2 tablespoons chopped unsalted dry-roasted peanuts (optional)

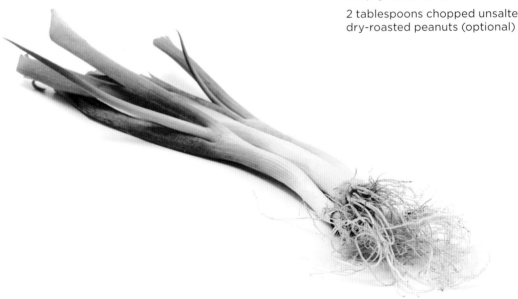

Per serving (with nuts): calories 90, total fat 4g, saturated fat 0.5g, cholesterol 0mg, sodium 155mg, carbohydrates 10g, dietary fiber 2g, sugars 3g, protein 3g
Percent Daily Value: vitamin A 189%, vitamin C 54%, iron 9%, calcium 9%

Just Call Me Baby Bok Choy

heart | can | bloat | skin | slim | stress | mood

This baby bok choy is so tender and delicate it will seduce even the toughest palates to please. Plus, your waistline will thank you, since it will help fill you for just 15 calories a serving! Whenever we have this for dinner, we crave the leftovers of this Asian-inspired dish at lunch.

Serves 4 (1 baby bok choy per serving)

4 washed baby bok choy (whole)

1 tablespoon low-sodium soy sauce

2 garlic cloves, crushed

1. Preheat oven to 350°F.

2. Spread whole bok choy evenly across a baking pan.

3. Drizzle with soy sauce and sprinkle with garlic.

4. Roast at 350°F for 20 minutes or until the bok choy are tender and the leaves have started to wilt.

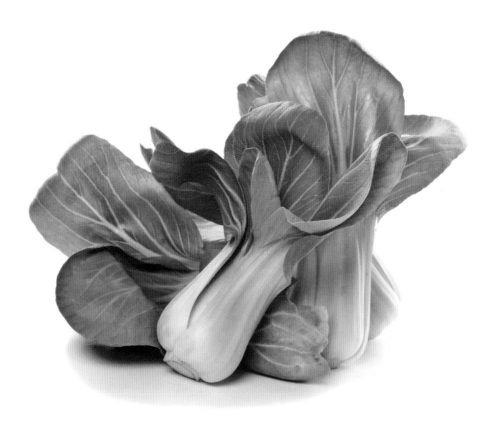

Per serving: calories 15, total fat 0g, saturated fat 0g, cholesterol 0g, sodium 134mg, carbohydrates 3g, dietary fiber 1g, sugars 0g, protein 2g
Percent Daily Value: vitamin A 119%, vitamin C 61%, calcium 9%, iron 9%

Oh Baby! Brussels Sprouts

heart | can | full

Whether you are preparing these with baby brussels sprouts or simply using these "baby" cabbages, they'll make your taste buds sing. They are so yummy and easy to make, they'll likely become a regular in your house, like they are in ours.

Serves 2 (1¼ cups per serving)

1. Preheat oven to 425°F.

2. Prepare the frozen vegetables according to package directions and drain excess liquid. If using fresh, put sprouts in a microwave-safe bowl and add 1 to 2 inches of water. Cover the bowl and cook on high for approximately 5 minutes. (Microwave cooking times will vary, depending on the size and quantity of the sprouts. You may need an additional 1 to 5 minutes to reach the preferred tenderness.)

3. In a small baking dish or gratin dish, spray the brussels sprouts with butter spray and season with black pepper.

4. Roast for 15 minutes. Remove from the oven, stir the sprouts, and sprinkle with cheese. Roast for another 10 minutes. Serve.

Variation: If you are extremely hurried or trying to cut calories, simply leave out the last step. You'll have a yummy, buttery, low-calorie veggie ready in minutes. (You'll shave off about 22 calories and 75 milligrams of sodium.)

1 (12-ounce) bag fresh or frozen brussels sprouts, microwave steam bags preferred

15 sprays I Can't Believe It's Not Butter! spray

Freshly ground black pepper to taste

2 tablespoons finely shredded Parmesan cheese

> We've been using I Can't Believe It's Not Butter! spray for years because we love that it allows you to add a great buttery flavor to veggies without adding any calories or artery-clogging fat like you'd find in butter. It seems that a little bit goes a long way when helping people to enjoy their veggies.

Per serving: calories 101, total fat 3g, saturated fat 1g, cholesterol 4mg, sodium 103mg, carbohydrates 14g, dietary fiber 7g, sugars 0g, protein 8g
Percent Daily Value: vitamin A 22%, vitamin C 211%, iron 9%, calcium 10%

Potato Bites

heart | preg | can | kid | bloat | skin | energy | full | stress | mood | bones

We serve these (our version of crispy hash browns) with morning brunch or as a side with dinner. Either hour they're a crowd-pleaser and a great way to boost your energy. If you have kids, count them in.

Serves 4 (¾ cup per serving)

4 cups cubed potatoes

Cooking spray

2½ teaspoons garlic powder

2½ teaspoons onion powder

½ teaspoon paprika

2 teaspoons rosemary

¾ teaspoon black pepper

3 tablespoons Parmesan cheese

Salt and freshly ground pepper to taste (optional)

1. Preheat oven to 425°F.

2. Spread potatoes on a baking dish and lightly spray with cooking spray. Sprinkle garlic powder, onion powder, paprika, rosemary, black pepper, and Parmesan cheese onto potatoes. Toss potato cubes until they are evenly coated with seasonings and cheese.

3. Arrange the potatoes evenly on the baking dish and place in oven. Bake for 30 minutes.

4. Toss the potatoes and return dish to oven to bake for about 15 to 25 minutes more or until golden and crispy.

5. Add freshly ground pepper and salt to taste (if desired). Serve hot.

Per serving: calories 177, total fat 2g, saturated fat 1g, cholesterol 3mg, sodium 67mg, carbohydrates 37g, dietary fiber 3g, sugars 4g, protein 5g
Percent Daily Value: vitamin A 3%, vitamin C 35%, calcium 6%, iron 5%

Roasted Fennel

can | bloat | skin | stress | mood | detox

This recipe is so simple, yet so delicious. Roasting the fennel brings out its sweetness, and to us it's like candy. The Parmesan adds a lot of flavor for a small amount of calories.

Serves 6 (1 cup per serving)

1. Preheat the oven to 375°F.

2. With your fingers, oil a large glass baking dish with ½ teaspoon of olive oil.

3. In a large bowl, rub the fennel with the remaining 1 teaspoon of olive oil, pepper, and salt (if using). Layer the fennel in the prepared baking dish. Scatter the Parmesan on top and roast until the fennel is fork tender and the top is golden brown, about 60 minutes.

Tip: Use a microplane or the small-hole shredder side of your box grater for the Parmesan. This helps a little cheese go a long way.

1½ teaspoons extra-virgin olive oil, divided

4 fennel bulbs, cored and cut into thin (approximately ⅓-inch) slices

Freshly ground black pepper to taste

Salt to taste (optional)

¼ cup finely shredded Parmesan cheese

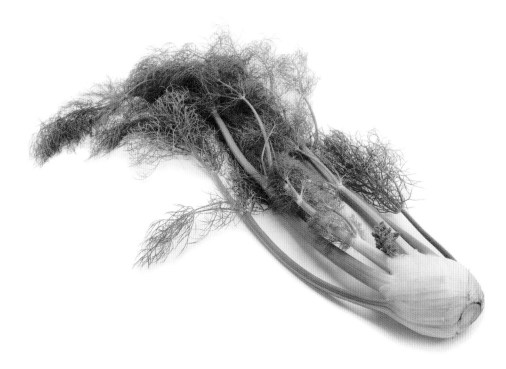

Per serving (without optional salt): calories 46, total fat 2g, saturated fat 1g, cholesterol 4mg, sodium 94mg, carbohydrates 4g, dietary fiber 2g, sugars 0g, protein 2g
Percent Daily Value: vitamin A 2%, vitamin C 12%, iron 3%, calcium 7%

Roasted Garlic Broccolini

heart | can | kid | skin | slim

This has been a staple in our family for years. It's quick and easy and makes a great veggie companion to fish, chicken, or pasta. The sweet and tender broccolini takes on a delicious garlicky flavor, and for 19 calories per half cup, you can't go wrong, as you could have five servings for fewer calories than a piece of bread! This recipe can be made with the entire broccolini spear, not just the florets.

Serves 4 (½ cup per serving)

2 cups broccolini florets

7–8 pumps I Can't Believe It's Not Butter! spray

1 small garlic clove, minced

Sprinkling of freshly ground black pepper

Sprinkling of oregano

Sprinkling of garlic powder

Sprinkling of red pepper flakes (optional)

1. Preheat oven or toaster oven to 425°F.

2. Line a baking tray with aluminum foil and lay the broccolini evenly across the tray.

3. Lightly spray broccolini with butter spray and sprinkle with garlic, pepper, oregano, garlic powder, and red pepper flakes (if using).

4. Place in the oven or toaster. Broccolini is ready when it starts to slightly turn a golden brown, about 8 to 10 minutes.

Tip: If you've never used butter spray before, you'll love that you can simply squirt it on your food and get all of the great buttery flavor, but without calories or artery-clogging fat.

Per serving: calories 19, total fat 0g, saturated fat 0g, cholesterol 0mg, sodium 20mg, carbohydrates 4g, dietary fiber 1g, sugars 1g, protein 1g
Percent Daily Value: vitamin A 0%, vitamin C 67%, calcium 4%, iron 4%

Savory Brussels Sprouts

heart | can

We love that these savory bites can be whipped up in minutes and shoved in the oven for less than a half hour, yet taste like you have spent hours preparing them. Plus, you can make these year-round—just buy the frozen variety. We favor the mini brussels sprouts, as they seem extra sweet. And for just 89 calories per serving, you'll fight cancer, heart disease, and aging—all in a delicious package that's always quickly devoured.

Serves 3 (1 cup per serving)

2 cups frozen or fresh mini brussels sprouts

1 8-ounce can sliced water chestnuts

½ cup low-sodium vegetable broth

¼–½ teaspoon freshly ground black pepper

1 tablespoon vegetarian bacon bits (optional)

1. Preheat oven to 375°F.

2. Place brussels sprouts in a casserole dish with water chestnuts.

3. Add broth and pepper and toss until evenly coated.

4. Bake for 25 minutes, turning the brussels sprouts once halfway through. Sprinkle with bacon bits (if desired).

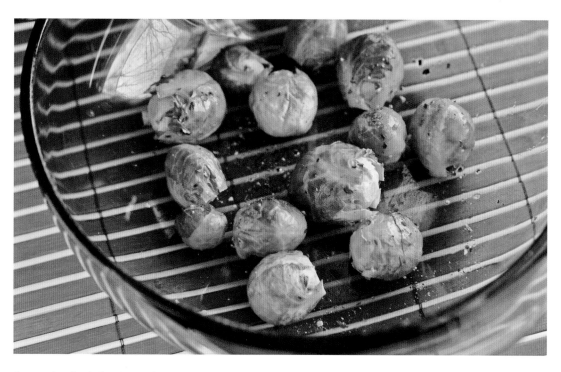

Per serving (including bacon bits): calories 89, total fat 1g, saturated fat 0g, sodium 69mg, dietary fiber 4g, carbohydrates 16g, sugars 2g, protein 6g
Percent Daily Value: vitamin A 20%, vitamin C 86%, calcium 3%, iron 4%

Simple Sautéed Spinach

heart | can | preg | bones | slim | bloat | skin | stress | mood | time

We love this dish because within minutes you can augment any meal with a delicious, low-calorie, nutrient-packed side that's as healthy as if it were simply steamed. Plus, it packs so much flavor that you'll want to eat more of it and less of the higher-calorie main dish.

Serves 4

Olive oil spray

1½ cloves garlic

4 cups chopped (4 ounces trimmed, mature leaves) spinach

1 tablespoon lemon juice

¼ teaspoon crushed red pepper

Salt to taste (optional)

1. Crush garlic and let it sit for 5 minutes to enhance its potent health-promoting antioxidants.

2. Spray frying pan with olive oil and add garlic. Sauté on medium heat for 1 minute, then add spinach and sauté for about another 3 minutes or until wilted.

3. Add lemon juice and crushed red pepper. Salt lightly (if desired) to taste.

Tip: For the spinach, you can substitute any leafy green you have on hand.

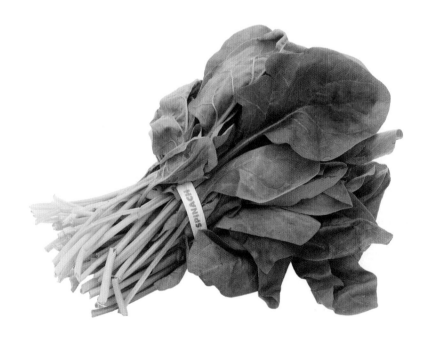

Per serving (without added salt): calories 38, total fat 0g, saturated fat 0g, cholesterol 0mg, sodium 96mg, carbohydrates 7g, dietary fiber 3g, sugars 1g, protein 4g
Percent Daily Value: vitamin A 225%, vitamin C 70%, calcium 13%, iron 18%

Slam, Bam, Thank You Ma'am 5-Minute Broccoli or Cauliflower

heart | preg | can | kid | slim | bloat | stress | mood | detox | skin | time

For a delish veggie in a jiffy, this is your ultimate go-to recipe. Defrost your broccoli or cauliflower in the fridge overnight, come home from work or from working out, drain, and toss one of our vinaigrettes on it. Bam! A scrumptious and soft-cooked veggie in moments is on your plate.

Serves 4 (approximately 1 cup per serving)

1. Defrost a bag of frozen broccoli and/or cauliflower overnight in the refrigerator.

2. Drain out the extra water and toss in our Herbed Vinaigrette (page 184) or Honey Dijon Vinaigrette (page 169) or your favorite light dressing.

3. Enjoy as a healthy side or snack!

Variation: You can use fresh broccoli or cauliflower, but it won't have the soft-cooked texture that defrosted vegetables have.

1 (16-ounce) bag frozen broccoli and/or cauliflower

4 tablespoons light salad dressing

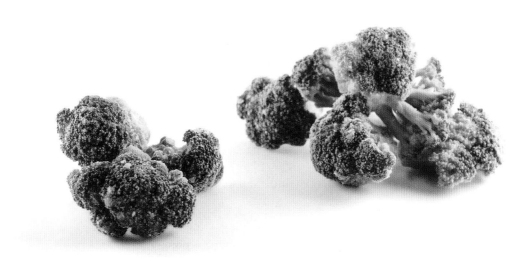

Per serving (with our Herbed Vinaigrette): calories 44, total fat 2g, saturated fat 9g, cholesterol 0mg, sodium 69mg, carbohydrates 6g, dietary fiber 3g, sugars 2g, protein 3g
Percent Daily Value: vitamin A 23%, vitamin C 106%, calcium 6%, iron 5%

Sriracha Potato Cha Cha

preg | can | kid | bloat | skin | energy | full | stress | mood

These potatoes are so good they'll make your taste buds and your entire body dance the cha-cha! We love these little bite-size potatoes, and so do the little ones. They'll give you an energy burst and spirit boost as well as a nice dose of fiber!

Serves 4 (½ cup per serving)

4 russet potatoes (about 5 ounces each), peeled and wrapped in aluminum foil

1 teaspoon sriracha hot sauce

2 tablespoons light butter-flavored spread made with vegetable oils

Salt to taste

1. Preheat oven to 400°F.

2. Roast the potatoes in the oven for 45 to 60 minutes or until very soft.

3. Place the hot potatoes in a heatproof bowl and mash thoroughly with a fork. Add the sriracha and vegetable spread. Mash until smooth and fluffy with a fork. Salt to taste. Serve.

Mix it up. Try some smoky heat. Replace the sriracha with half a dried chipotle pepper, stemmed, seeded, and ground fine into a powder in a coffee grinder or blender. Can't find dried chipotle peppers? Substitute 1 teaspoon of a chipotle hot sauce like Tabasco or Cholula brand for the dried pepper.

Per serving (without added salt): calories 158, total fat 3g, saturated fat 1g, cholesterol 0mg, sodium 87mg, carbohydrates 30g, dietary fiber 3g, sugars 2g, protein 4g
Percent Daily Value: vitamin A 5%, vitamin C 30%, iron 8%, calcium 2%

Teriyaki-Lime Veggie and Pineapple Kebabs

preg | can | slim | bloat | skin | stress | mood | kid | heart | bones

There's nothing like good food on a skewer, and this kebab takes the cake—or skewer! It will make your mouth water, thanks to the grilling that caramelizes the veggies and the pineapple that makes it taste like candy. Kids and adults alike will ask for this scrumptious mood-boosting dish. No one will ever believe it's actually good for them to boot!

Serves 4 (1 skewer per serving)

1. Preheat grill to medium-high.

2. Cut veggies and pineapple into chunks. Thread onto skewers.

3. Spray with olive oil spray.

4. Place kebabs on grill. Cook for 20 minutes, flipping the kebabs halfway through.

5. Once cooked, lightly brush kebabs with teriyaki glaze. Sprinkle with lime juice. Add pepper to taste.

4 flexible (kid-friendly) skewers

1 red bell pepper

1 orange bell pepper

1 small zucchini

1 small yellow squash

1 small white onion

1 cup pineapple

Olive oil cooking spray

1 tablespoon low-sodium teri-yaki glaze

Juice of 1 lime

Freshly ground black pepper

If you don't have a grill or prefer to stay inside in the colder months, this recipe works just as well broiling the veggies! Broil on high and the cooking times will be the same. If you don't have skewers, you can make these veggies on a baking pan that has been sprayed with cooking spray.

Per serving: calories 75, total fat 1g, saturated fat 0g, cholesterol 0g, sodium 69mg, carbohydrates 15g, dietary fiber 3g, sugars 8g, protein 2g
Percent Daily Value: vitamin A 23%, vitamin C 263%, calcium 3%, iron 4%

The Nutrition Twins' Skinny Cauliflower Mash

heart | preg | can | kid | slim | bloat | stress | mood | detox

This recipe is the perfect "lightened up" version of mashed potatoes. Your family won't even notice it's not the real deal. You can modify it for your taste—more garlicky, more tangy with lemon. However you choose, it will still be a low-calorie, scrumptious mashed potato alternative that fights heart disease, cancer, and the blues.

Serves 3 (about ¾ cup per serving)

1 (16-ounce bag) bag frozen cauliflower

½ teaspoon (1 small clove) garlic

⅛ cup skim milk

1 teaspoon dried chives (optional)

Freshly ground black pepper to taste

½ teaspoon lemon juice (optional)

1. Defrost cauliflower in the microwave or overnight in the refrigerator.

2. Crush garlic and let it sit for 5 minutes to release its health-promoting properties.

3. Place cauliflower in a blender or food processor along with milk, garlic, chives (if using), and pepper.

4. Add lemon juice (if using) and sample for taste. Add more garlic, lemon, chives, or pepper as desired.

Tip: If you want to use fresh cauliflower, simply substitute 1 medium head for the frozen 1-pound bag, steam it or cook it in the microwave, and then begin with step 2.

Per serving: calories 43, total fat 0g, saturated fat 0g, cholesterol 0mg, sodium 46mg, carbohydrates 8g, dietary fiber 3g, sugars 4g, protein 4g
Percent Daily Value: vitamin A 1%, vitamin C 123%, calcium 6%, iron 5%

Vegetable Ribbons

kid | slim | skin | detox | preg | stress | mood

This dish not only tastes great but looks really pretty with hardly any effort. Kids love eating the ribbons that look like they were slaved over yet were actually prepared in just minutes! So sit back, enjoy, and let the nutrients in the "ribbons" relax you as they give you a "facial" and beautify your skin from the inside out.

Serves 4 (½ cup per serving)

1. Scrub carrots and zucchini; cut off ends. Use a peeler to create ribbons by holding the vegetables down on a cutting board while peeling and rotating every so often.

2. Heat the oil in a large skillet over medium heat. (Or lightly coat pan with cooking spray.) Add the vegetable ribbons, stir, cover with a tight-fitting lid, and cook for 3 to 4 minutes or until vegetables are tender but not overcooked.

3. Remove from heat, add pepper and salt (if desired), and serve immediately.

1 large carrot

1 medium zucchini

1 teaspoon olive or vegetable oil (or oil in spray bottle)

¼ teaspoon freshly ground black pepper (optional)

Dash of salt (optional)

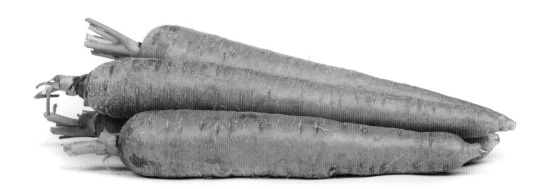

Per serving (with 1 teaspoon olive oil and no salt): calories 24, total fat 1g, saturated fat 0g, cholesterol 0mg, sodium 15mg, carbohydrates 3g, dietary fiber 1g, sugars 2g, protein 1g
Percent Daily Value: vitamin A 53%, vitamin C 15%, calcium 1%, iron 1%

10-Day Weight Loss Jumpstart, Belly De-Bloat, and Toxin Flush

You now know that vegetables hold the power to keep every part of your body in better working order—and to help your body to achieve its optimal level of health and wellness.

Vegetables can maximize your energy, fend off disease, help keep your body youthful, slim you down, and accentuate your beauty. Let this 10-Day Jumpstart be your guide to help you to get the most out of your Veggie Cure weight loss prescription.

Below you will see a list of bulleted guidelines for your 10-Day Jumpstart. Although by simply following the menu plan (page 242), you will be adhering to many of these recommendations that will help you to realize your ultimate weight loss, de-bloating, and toxin-flushing potential, be sure to read the tips below. They will guide you in the process and are good habits to create for a lifetime of lean and healthy living. If for any reason you are unable to follow the menu plan to a tee, be sure to stick to these recommendations and use the menu as a guide to help you in your 10-day detox.

Note: If you've overdone it with too much food and drink and/or not enough exercise and now feel tired, waterlogged, heavy, bloated—or you are experiencing swollen hands and feet, puffiness under your eyes, constipation, or a headache—this 10-day flush will bring an abrupt end to many of these symptoms. It will also immediately get your body and mind back on the healthy track.

- Start each day by drinking 16 ounces of water and either our Minted Mango Melon Detox Smoothie (page 111), Green Minted Cocoa Detox Smoothie (page 110), or Berry Yogurt Detox Smoothie (page 106) to hydrate and start the day by flooding your body with antioxidants. If you choose to have two servings of one of these detox smoothies, you can start the day by drinking 8 ounces of water instead of 16.

- Drink 16 ounces of water, green tea, Sparkling Cucumber Detox and Refresher (page 113), or a combination totaling 16 ounces of any at meals, excluding breakfast.

- Follow our "Red, Green, and Orange Rule": Include a "red," "orange," or "green" type of produce (fruit or vegetable) at every meal. By choosing any of our recipes at mealtimes, you will automatically do this.

- Whenever you feel hungry, whether after a meal or snack, fill up on vegetables, raw or steamed plain with spices, lemon, or flavored vinegars. Or go for our ultralow-calorie recipes like Slam, Bam, Thank You Ma'am 5-Minute Broccoli or Cauliflower (page 235), Cool Cucumber Bites (page 211), Roasted Turnip Nips (page 151), Bengali Cabbage (page 205), or Guilt-Free Kale Chips (page 143). As an alternative, you also can drink the Sparkling Cucumber Detox and Refresher (page 113) to tide you over for a bit.

- If you are looking to eat more of something, non-starchy vegetables are your ticket. Feel free to include more than the menu plans list.

- At meals, your plate should be composed of one-half vegetables.

- Choose organic foods when possible.

- Avoid alcoholic beverages.

- Steer clear of fried foods.

- Avoid fatty meats such as bacon, sausage, and veal, and meats that contain the known carcinogens nitrates/nitrites.

- Limit refined sugars (high-fructose corn syrup, corn syrup, honey, etc.) by choosing fruits for desserts rather than cakes, cookies, ice cream, candies, and candy bars—or limit any of these options to 100 calories or less daily.

- Refrain from adding salt at the table.

- Choose whole grains instead of white, refined breads, pastas, and rice. Limit to one cup or less per meal.

- If you are unable to eat a meal listed on the menu plan, be sure to get protein at each meal. Choose either a half cup of beans, tempeh, or tofu; 3 ounces of fish or poultry breast; 3 ounces of lean beef (maximum of twice per week); one egg or four to five egg whites; 6 ounces of nonfat yogurt; 1.5 ounces of low-fat or nonfat cheese; one cup of nonfat milk; half a cup of low-fat cottage cheese; two tablespoons nuts or seeds; or one tablespoon nut butter.

- Exercise daily, aiming for a minimum of 30 minutes each day and ideally one hour.

- Chew your food slowly and savor your meal. This will help you to enjoy it, feel satisfied, and prevent belly-bloat from overeating and swallowing air, both of which happen when you eat quickly.

Please note that this 10-Day Jumpstart is a low-calorie diet, averaging about 1,200 calories each day. Men and some very active women may need to increase snacks and/or have an extra half serving at some meals if they are losing weight too quickly. And if this plan is right for you but you find yourself feeling overly hungry, remember the key: Take every opportunity to include extra vegetables, raw or steamed plain, and fill up on non-starchy ones.

Note: Vegans and vegetarians can replace dairy products with protein- and calcium-rich nondairy alternatives.

Menus

	DAY 1	DAY 2
Breakfast	16 ounces water Berry Yogurt Detox Smoothie (p. 106) 1 slice whole wheat toast with 1 teaspoon peanut butter and 1 teaspoon low-sugar jam **OR** 8 ounces water 2 servings Berry Yogurt Detox Smoothie (p. 106)	16 ounces water Minted Mango Melon Detox Smoothie (p. 111) 2 Beet and Carrot Savory Pancakes (p. 114) **OR** 8 ounces water 2 servings Minted Mango Melon Detox Smoothie (p. 111)* (*If you choose this option, have ½ cup Artichoke Hummus [p. 126] or an extra half banana at snacktime)
Lunch	Asian Lettuce Wrap with Hoisin-Ginger Dipping Sauce (p. 170)	Tomato, Spinach, Egg 'n' Feta Never Tasted Betta Wrap (p. 123) 1 apple or other piece of fruit
Snack	Sparkling Cucumber Detox and Refresher (p. 113) 30 pistachios	2 servings Artichoke Hummus (p. 126) 8 whole wheat crackers **OR** Hard-boiled egg Half a banana
Dinner	Tomato and Basil Bruschetta (p. 157) Cauliflower Crusted Mozzarella Pie (p. 186)	Eggplant Parmesan (p. 187)
Snack	Green Minted Cocoa Detox Smoothie (p. 110) 1 nonfat Greek yogurt	1 cup green tea Low-fat string cheese 1 apple

	DAY 3	DAY4
Breakfast	16 ounces water Berry Yogurt Detox Smoothie (p. 106) Hole-in-One (p. 116) **OR** 8 ounces water 2 servings Berry Yogurt Detox Smoothie (p. 106)	16 ounces water Green Minted Cocoa Detox Smoothie (p. 110) Pumpkin 'n' Apple-y Yogurt Parfait (p. 118) **OR** 8 ounces water 2 servings Green Minted Cocoa Detox Smoothie (p. 110)* (*If you choose this option, have an additional half serving Zucchinilicious Lasagna [p. 204] at lunch or a string cheese. Otherwise, be sure to choose the parfait for your afternoon snack.
Lunch	Dieter's Delight Chock Full of Veggie Soup (p. 163) Cheese toast: 1 ounce low-fat cheese melted on 1 slice whole grain bread	2 servings Zucchinilicious Lasagna (p. 204)
Snack	Carrot Zucchini Muffin (p. 128) Sparkling Cucumber Detox and Refresher (p. 113) **OR** 1 cup carrot and zucchini slices dipped in ¼ cup Artichoke Hummus (p. 126) or store-bought hummus, or ⅔ cup shelled edamame	½ cup blueberries 1 cup green tea Minted Mango Melon Detox Smoothie (p. 111) **OR** Pumpkin 'n' Apple-y Yogurt Parfait (p. 118)
Dinner	Spaghetti Squash with Fresh Tomato Sauce (p. 200) Rockin' Ratatouille (p. 152) Roasted Garlic Broccolini (p. 232)	Stuffed Peppers (p. 202) Jicama Fried Rice (p. 226)
Snack	Trail mix: ¼ cup raisins, 2 tablespoons almonds Sparkling Cucumber Detox and Refresher (p. 113, optional)	Butternut Squash and Mango Mash (p. 210)

Menus

	DAY 5	DAY 6
Breakfast	16 ounces water Berry Yogurt Detox Smoothie (p. 106) 2 servings Veggie Frittata Bites (p. 121) **OR** 8 ounces water 2 servings Berry Yogurt Detox Smoothie (p. 106)	16 ounces water Berry Yogurt Detox Smoothie (p. 106) Tomato, Spinach, Egg 'n' Feta Never Tasted Betta Wrap (p. 123) **OR** 8 ounces water 2 servings Berry Yogurt Detox Smoothie (p. 106)
Lunch	I Beg Your Parsnips (p. 146) Sweet Potato Veggie burgers (p. 203)	Swiss Chard Salad with Red and Golden Beets and Honey Yogurt Vinaigrette (p. 182) Cold Cucumber and Avocado Soup (p. 160)
Snack	1 orange 30 pistachios Sparkling Cucumber Detox and Refresher (p. 113)	Spinach Squares (p. 154) Sparkling Cucumber Detox and Refresher (p. 113) **OR** ⅓ cup shelled edamame or a hard-boiled egg Sparkling Cucumber Detox and Refresher (p. 113)
Dinner	Heavenly Roasted Veggies (p. 219) 3 servings Roasted Red Pepper, Spinach, and Feta Portobello Burger (p. 196)	Roasted Tomato Puttanesca (p. 199) with 1 cup whole wheat pasta
Snack	Green Minted Cocoa Detox Smoothie (p. 110) ½ cup berries	6 ounces nonfat Greek yogurt 2 tablespoons walnut pieces 1 peach or other piece of fruit

	DAY 7	DAY 8
Breakfast	16 ounces water Minted Mango Melon Detox Smoothie (p. 111) Zucchini Fritters (p. 124) **OR** 8 ounces water 2 servings Minted Mango Melon Detox Smoothie (p. 111)* (*Have a hard-boiled egg with your snack or ½ cup cooked oatmeal or quinoa with breakfast or snack)	16 ounces water Green Minted Cocoa Detox Smoothie (p. 110) 2 servings Sweet and Savory Pumpkin Quiche (p. 120) **OR** 8 ounces water 2 servings Green Minted Cocoa Detox Smoothie (p. 110)* (*Have an extra half serving of Red Cabbage Salad with Grapes and Ginger Dressing [p. 180] at lunch or have 15 pistachios with your snack)
Lunch	Mediterranean Pizza (p. 192) 1 cup strawberries	Sweet Potato Veggie Burgers (p. 203) Red Cabbage Salad with Grapes and Ginger Dressing (p. 180)
Snack	2 servings Guilt-Free Kale Chips (p. 143) **OR** 2 servings Roasted Turnip Nips (p. 151) Sparkling Cucumber Detox and Refresher (p. 113)	2 servings Cool Cucumber Bites (p. 211)
Dinner	Stuffed Celery Bites (p. 155) Fennel Stuffed Potatoes (p. 189)	Arugula Salad with Strawberry Rhubarb Vinaigrette (p. 168) 2 cups Split Pea and Barley Soup (p. 166)
Snack	2 Pumpkin Cream Cheese Muffins (p. 149)	Minted Mango Melon Detox Smoothie (p. 111)

Menus

	DAY 9	DAY 10
Beakfast	16 ounces of water Minted Mango Melon Detox Smoothie (p. 111) Cheese toast: 1 slice whole grain toast with 1 ounce nonfat cheese 1 slice tomato **OR** 8 ounces water 2 Servings Minted Mango Melon Detox Smoothie (p. 111)	16 ounces water Green Minted Cocoa Detox Smoothie (p. 110) 2 servings Veggie Frittata Bites (p. 121) **OR** 8 ounces water 2 servings Green Minted Cocoa Detox Smoothie (p. 110)
Lunch	Tomato Artichoke Pasta Bake (p. 201)	Quinoa with Mixed Vegetables (p. 193) Chipotle Smashed Sweet Potatoes (p. 212)
Snack	Curried Sweet Potato and Apple Salad (p. 132)	Edamame and Corn Salad (p. 173) Sparkling Cucumber Detox and Refresher (p. 113)
Dinner	Green Bean Salad with Toasted Almonds and Dates (p. 218) 2 cups Hot Diggity Chili (p. 195)	Ole! Mexican Cabbage with Black Beans and Avocados (p. 179)
Snack	Cheese and berry plate: 1 ounce low-fat cheese, ½ cup mixed berries	Minted Mango Melon Detox Smoo[...] (p. 111) 1 apple

Metric Conversion Tables

METRIC/U.S. APPROXIMATE EQUIVALENTS

Liquid Ingredients

METRIC	U.S. MEASURES	METRIC	U.S. MEASURES
1.23 ML	¼ TSP.	29.57 ML	2 TBSP.
2.36 ML	½ TSP.	44.36 ML	3 TBSP.
3.70 ML	¾ TSP.	59.15 ML	¼ CUP
4.93 ML	1 TSP.	118.30 ML	½ CUP
6.16 ML	1¼ TSP.	236.59 ML	1 CUP
7.39 ML	1½ TSP.	473.18 ML	2 CUPS OR 1 PT.
8.63 ML	1¾ TSP.	709.77 ML	3 CUPS
9.86 ML	2 TSP.	946.36 ML	4 CUPS OR 1 QT.
14.79 ML	1 TBSP.	3.791L	4 QTS. OR 1 GAL.

Dry Ingredients

METRIC	U.S. MEASURES	METRIC	U.S. MEASURES
2 (1.8) G	1/16 OZ.	80 G	2⅘ OZ.
3½ (3.5) G	⅛ OZ.	85 (84.9) G	3 OZ.
7 (7.1) G	¼ OZ.	100 G	3½ OZ.
15 (14.2) G	½ OZ.	115 (113.2) G	4 OZ.
21 (21.3) G	¾ OZ.	125 G	4½ OZ.
25 G	⅞ OZ.	150 G	5¼ OZ.
30 (28.3) G	1 OZ.	250 G	8⅞ OZ.
50 G	1¾ OZ.	454 G	1 LB. 16 OZ.
60 (56.6) G	2 OZ.	500 G	1 LIVRE 17⅗ OZ.

Acknowledgments

A heartfelt thanks to all of the people who have helped us to bring this book to the shelves.

To our outstanding literary agent, Laura Dail, of Laura Dail Literary Agency, for always believing in us, encouraging us, and for working your magic to make this all happen. We trust you and value your opinion more than you'll ever know.

Special thanks to our fabulous editor, Mary Norris. You are an absolute dream to work with, and we can't thank you enough for your hard work and dedication. Even through e-mails we could feel your sweet energy guiding us with a smile.

Our warmest thanks to everyone at Globe Pequot Press, especially to David Legere and Meredith Dias for guiding this book through to its finish; to Diana Nuhn for your wonderful design creativity. Thanks also to copyeditor Ann Marlowe, proofreader Ann Seifert, and indexer Jan Mucciarone.

Thank you to Stephanie for your stunningly beautiful food styling, your gorgeous photos, and your incredibly helpful recipe feedback.

Thanks to the amazing Carol Gelles. It was an absolute thrill to work with the culinary crème de la crème. Your prowess in the kitchen amazes us, and your ability to conceptualize recipes is extraordinary. We are honored and humbled to have a James Beard and Julia Child award–winning chef's innovative vegetarian recipes created for our book. Thank you for being our beloved mother hen, sharing your expertise and guiding us through the recipe webs.

And to the fantastic Joe Landa, we are so grateful for your scrumptious creations and are in awe of your fabulous Beethoven-like ability to turn random ingredients into masterpieces. We are thrilled to have the winner of Food Network's *Chopped* creating strokes of genius for us. Without your recipe contributions, this book would not be what it is. You have tantalized our taste buds, and we can't wait for the world to try your inventions.

Many thanks to Jake Fontanilla for your tasty contributions. And to Sharon Palmer, our fabulous veggie-loving friend and registered dietitian, for yours.

To our incredible research intern, Katie Andrews—for your savvy and critical eye, we are forever grateful.

To our smart and hardworking intern Morgan Deihs, thank you for dedicating your valuable time and for lending your culinary skills for the marketing of this book. You are a force to be reckoned with and are going to continue to shine in the nutrition world.

To our fabulous interns Jo Ann Brown, Veronica Sommer, and Bonnie Averbach, you ladies were true rock stars.

Thanks to you and our other hardworking interns—Francesca Dell'olio, Samantha Bernstein, Miriam Raskin, Dassy Levilev, Eden Goykadosh, Pui Lun Christin Chan, Adrian Hernandez, Olena Gudz, Morgan Blonder, and Katie Leonard— for your dedication and help with recipe trial and error and nutrient analysis. We're proud to have had you with us. All of you are going to make fantastic dietitians, and we look forward to following your paths and learning of your accomplishments.

Thank you to our clients and social media followers who motivated us to write this book. Your e-mails, letters, and phone calls explaining how our veggie recipes have improved your health, changed your lives, and made you start craving veggies and more vegetable recipes was the inspiration we needed to write this book.

To Laura Lockwood and Libby Isaacman, whose creative cooking served as an inspiration. A humongous embrace and thanks for keeping us creative and for helping us to find tasty ways to spice up any dish.

A huge hug to you, Mom. We are so grateful to you for serving us nutrient-rich veggies every night while growing up. Thank you and Dad, too, for setting such a healthy example. We greatly admire you for your persistence and for not backing down when we'd try to avoid eating them. Because of your consistency, we ultimately embraced vegetables and don't go a day without a lot of them. And thanks to both of you for your love and support in everything that we do—without you both, we would never be where we are today.

And our most profound thanks goes to both Tammy's husband, Scott, and Lyssie's boyfriend, Darren: Thank you for your constant support and for your patience and understanding with the long hours of writing. We are both now available to play. Phew! We are so grateful for your love and support throughout this process and throughout the days of our lives together.

Last, but certainly not least, thanks to Tammy's twin daughters, Summer and Riley, for being guinea pigs and allowing us to test our kid concoctions on you. You always make us happy after a long day. We love you very much.

Recipe Index

Appetizers and Snacks

Artichoke Hummus, 126
Carrot Zucchini Muffins, 128
Cauliflower Ceviche, 127
Coco Sweet Potatoes with Mango
    Salsa, 130
Corn and Bean Salsa, 131
Creamy Spinach Dip, 134
Curried Sweet Potato and Apple
    Salad, 132
Fig and Olive Tapenade, 135
Garlic and Herb Potato Stacks, 136
Golden Gazpacho in Petite Cucumber
    Cradles, 139
Green Pea Hummus, 137
Guacamole Stuffed Tomato Poppers, 140
Guilt-Free Kale Chips, 143
Holy Fruity Guacamole!, 144
I Beg Your Parsnips, 146
Muuuhr Muhammara Please, 145
Parmesan Baked Artichoke, 148
Pumpkin Cream Cheese Muffins, 149
Ribb—it! Frogs on a Celery-Rib Log, 150
Roasted Turnip Nips, 151
Rockin' Ratatouille, 152
Savory Sweet Potato Fries, 153
Spinach Squares, 154
Stuffed Celery Bites, 155
Tomato and Basil Bruschetta, 157
Zucchini Canoes, 158

Breakfasts and Smoothies

Beet and Carrot Savory Pancakes, 114
Berry Yogurt Detox Smoothie, 106
Cauliflower and Broccoli Flapjacks, 115
Fruity Green Smoothie, 108
Green Minted Cocoa Detox Smoothie, 110

Greenana Apple Pear Smoothie, 109
Hole-in-One, 116
Minted Mango Melon Detox Smoothie, 111
Pumpkin 'n' Apple-y Yogurt Parfait, 118
Pumpkin Pancakes, 117
Sparkling Cucumber Detox and
    Refresher, 113
Sweet and Savory Pumpkin Quiche, 120
Tomato, Spinach, Egg 'n' Feta Never Tasted
    Betta Wrap, 123
Veggie Frittata Bites, 121
Zucchini Fritters, 124

Main Dishes

Butternut and Turnip Barley Risotto, 185
Cauliflower Crusted Mozzarella Pie, 186
Eggplant Parmesan, 187
Fennel Stuffed Potatoes, 189
Grab and Go Pita Slaw Sandwich, 190
Hot Diggity Chili!, 195
Mediterranean Pizza, 192
Quinoa with Mixed Vegetables, 193
Roasted Red Pepper, Spinach, and Feta
    Portobello Burger, 196
Roasted Tomato Puttanesca, 199
Spaghetti Squash with Fresh Tomato
    Sauce, 200
Stuffed Peppers, 202
Sweet Potato Veggie Burgers, 203
Tomato Artichoke Pasta Bake, 201
Zucchinilicious Lasagna, 204

Side Dishes

Baby Bellas and Asparagus, 206
Bangin' Broccoli East Meets West
    Style, 209
Bengali Cabbage, 205

Butternut Squash and Mango Mash, 210

Chipotle Smashed Sweet Potatoes, 212

Cool Cucumber Bites, 211

Easy Spinach Pomodoro, 214

Floating Asparagus Rafts, 215

Green Bean Salad with Toasted Dates and Almonds, 218

Green Beans with Lemon Caper Vinaigrette, 217

Heavenly Roasted Vegetables, 219

Herb and Garlic Creamed Spinach, 220

Honey Ginger Carrot Coins, 223

Italian Mushrooms, Tomato, and Spinach, 224

Jicama Fried Rice, 226

Just Call Me Baby Bok Choy, 228

Kung Pao Veggies, 227

The Nutrition Twins' Skinny Cauliflower Mash, 238

Oh Baby! Brussels Sprouts, 229

Potato Bites, 230

Roasted Fennel, 231

Roasted Garlic Broccolini, 232

Savory Brussels Sprouts, 233

Simple Sautéed Spinach, 234

Slam, Bam, Thank You Ma'am 5-Minute Broccoli or Cauliflower, 235

Sriracha Potato Cha Cha, 236

Teriyaki-Lime Veggie and Pineapple Kebabs, 237

Vegetable Ribbons, 239

Soups and Salads

Arugula Salad with Strawberry Rhubarb Vinaigrette, 168

Asian Lettuce Wrap with Hoisin-Ginger Dipping Sauce, 170–71

Cold Cucumber and Avocado Soup, 160

Colorful Crunch Salad with Honey Dijon Vinaigrette, 169

Cream of Whatever Soup, 159

Dieter's Delight Chock Full of Veggies Soup, 163

Edamame and Corn Salad, 173

Grapefruit, Avocado, and Kale Salad with Pepitas, 174

Herbed Pea Soup with Spinach, 165

Herbed Romaine with Pine Nuts, 176

Herbed Vinaigrette, 184

Hickory Broccoli Salad, 175

Mojito Salad, 178

Ole! Mexican Cabbage with Black Beans and Avocados, 179

Red Cabbage Salad with Grapes and Ginger Dressing, 180

Refreshing Beet and Watermelon Detox Salad, 181

Split Pea and Barley Soup, 166

Swiss Chard Salad with Red and Golden Beets and Honey Yogurt Vinaigrette, 182

Vegetable Broth, 164

Veggie Yard Dash Salad, 183

Index

alpha-carotene, 70, 98

amines, 29, 67

anthocyanins, 18, 19, 72, 78, 84

artichokes, 8, 11–12, 17, 33, 34, 148

asparagus
>for bone health, 33
>for detoxing and cleansing, 76
>for heart disease, 15, 17
>for mood boosting, 65, 66
>for pregnancy, 55–57
>for stress and tension, 2
>vitamins and minerals, 2, 15, 17, 33, 55, 56, 57, 65, 66

avocados, 15, 17, 96–98, 140, 144

beans, 2, 3, 15, 17–19, 32, 34, 66

beet greens, 32–33, 34

beets, 15, 17, 76–79

bell peppers
>for bloating and constipation, 8
>cooking method, 100
>for heart disease, 15
>for mood boosting, 65, 66
>and paprika, 100
>for stress and tension, 2
>vitamins and minerals, 2, 8, 15, 65, 66, 99–100
>for weight loss, 39

beta-carotene, 50, 51–52, 64, 90, 92, 98

beta-cryptoxanthin, 70, 84

betalain, 76, 77, 78

blackstrap molasses, 15

bloating and constipation, 8–12

bok choy (Chinese cabbage)
>for bloating and constipation, 2, 26, 32, 33, 39–42, 76
>for bone health, 32, 33
>for cancer, 26, 42
>for detoxing and cleansing, 76
>for stress and tension, 2
>vitamins and minerals, 2, 33, 40, 41–42, 76
>for weight loss, 39–42

bone health, 31–38

broccoli
>for bloating and constipation, 8
>for bone health, 32
>for cancer, 26
>cooking method, 89, 91
>for detoxing and cleansing, 76
>for heart disease, 15, 17, 21
>kid-friendly veggies, 87, 89–91
>for mood boosting, 65, 66
>for stress and tension, 2
>vitamins and minerals, 2, 15, 17, 21, 32, 65, 66, 76, 90–91
>for weight loss, 39

brussels sprouts
>for bloating and constipation, 8
>for bone health, 33
>for cancer, 26, 29–30
>for detoxing and cleansing, 76
>for heart disease, 15, 17, 30
>for mood boosting, 66
>vitamins and minerals, 8, 17, 30, 33, 66, 76

cabbage (green, red, and savoy)
>for bloating and constipation, 8, 42
>for cancer, 26, 42
>for detoxing and cleansing, 76
>for heart disease, 15, 42
>for mood boosting, 66
>for stress and tension, 2
>vitamins and minerals, 2, 15, 40, 41–42, 76
>for weight loss, 39–42

calcium
    for bone health, 7, 10, 32, 34–35, 37–38
    for detoxing and cleansing, 80
    for pregnancy, 55, 57, 58
    for stress and tension, 2, 7
    for weight loss, 41, 43
cancer, 26–30
carotenoids and flavanoids
    for bone health, 7
    for cancer, 28
    for diabetes, 7
    for energy, 49
    for eye health, 5
    for heart disease, 7, 18, 19, 21
    for inflammatory diseases, 7
    for mood boosting, 68
    in salads, 83, 86
    for the skin, 53–54
carrots
    cooking, 90
    for detoxing and cleansing, 76
    for heart disease, 15, 17
    kid-friendly veggies, 87, 91–92
    for mood boosting, 66
    vitamins and minerals, 15, 17, 76, 92
    for weight loss, 39
cauliflower
    for bloating and constipation, 8
    for cancer, 26
    for detoxing and cleansing, 76
    for heart disease, 8, 17
    kid-friendly veggies, 87
    for mood boosting, 66
    for quick cooking, 60–62
    vitamins and minerals, 8, 15, 17, 62
    for weight loss, 39
collard greens, 2, 32, 33, 34, 66
copper, 2, 35, 37, 46, 74, 78
corn, 44, 65, 66, 82–84
cucumbers
    for bloating and constipation, 8

    and collagen, 54
    for detoxing and cleansing, 75
    for heart disease, 15, 17
    for the skin, 52–54
    for stress and tension, 2
    vitamins and minerals, 2, 8, 15, 17, 53, 54, 75
    for weight loss, 39
dandelion greens, 2, 32
dark leafy greens, 2, 8, 17, 32, 33, 39, 65
detox and cleanse, 75–80
edamame, 2, 95
eggplant, 15, 66, 71–73
energy – the perk-up factor, 44–49
fast foods, 13
fennel, 2, 8, 9–11, 15, 39, 76
fiber
    for bloating and constipation, 8, 10, 11
    for bone health, 32, 33
    for cancer, 28, 29, 36
    for cravings and overeating, 2
    for detoxing and cleansing, 75, 76, 78, 79, 80
    for diabetes, 36
    for digestive health, 30, 36
    for energy, 45, 47, 48
    for heart disease, 15, 16, 17, 18, 22, 30, 59
    for mood boosting, 65, 67, 68, 69
    for pregnancy, 55, 58, 59
    in salads, 82–83, 84
    for satisfying hunger, 72, 74
    for stress and tension, 2
    for weight loss, 40, 42, 43
folic acid (folate)
    for bloating and constipation, 10
    for cancer, 28–30, 36
    and common medications, 3
    for detoxing and cleansing, 78, 80, 83
    for energy, 47
    for heart disease, 16–17, 19, 22

for mood boosting, 65, 66, 69
for pregnancy, 55, 56, 57, 58
for satisfying hunger, 74
for stress and tension, 2, 4
for weight loss, 41
frozen, canned, and pre-chopped vegetables,
60–64, 104
garlic
for bone health, 33
for cancer, 26
for heart disease, 15, 23–25
for mood boosting, 66
preparing and cooking, 25, 104
and thiosulfinates, sulfoxides, dithiins,
and ajoene, 23
vitamins and minerals, 15, 25,
33, 66
glucosinolates, 26, 38, 90
heart disease and the cardiovascular system,
14–15
homocysteine levels, 16, 20, 25
iron, 7, 10, 55, 57, 58, 74, 78, 80
kale
for bone health, 32, 33
for cancer, 26
for detoxing and cleansing, 76, 79–80
for heart disease, 15, 21
for mood boosting, 66
for stress and tension, 2
vitamins and minerals, 2, 15, 21, 32, 33,
64, 66, 76, 79–80
for weight loss, 39
kid-friendly veggies, 87–89
leeks, 26, 33, 103
lettuce
for bloating and constipation, 8
for bone health, 33
for cancer, 26
for detoxing and cleansing, 76
for heart disease, 15
and obesity, 58
for pregnancy, 55

romaine lettuce, 57–59, 66
for stress and tension, 2
vitamins and minerals, 55–59, 76
lutein, 5, 64, 70, 98, 100, 160
lycopene, 32, 51, 52, 94, 96, 178
magnesium
for bone health, 7, 10, 32, 34, 35, 38
for detoxing and cleansing, 78, 80
for energy, 47
for heart disease, 19
for mood boosting, 70
for satisfying hunger, 72
for the skin, 54
for stress and tension, 2
for weight loss, 43
manganese
for bone health, 10, 12, 35, 38
for detoxing and cleansing, 78, 80
for heart disease, 21, 25
in salads, 84
for satisfying hunger, 72, 74
for the skin, 54
for weight loss, 41
Mediterranean diet, 34
melatonin, 67
microplanes, 103–4
molybdenum, 10, 100
mood-boosting veggies, 65–70
mushrooms
for bloating and constipation, 8
cooking methods, 21
crimini mushrooms (baby bella), 19–21,
65–66, 82–84
for detoxing and cleansing, 76
for heart disease, 15, 17–21
maitake mushrooms, 33
for mood boosting, 65–66
portobello, 20, 65
shiitake mushrooms, 15, 66
storing, 20–21
for stress and tension, 2
and ultraviolet light, 33

vitamins and nutrients, 2, 15, 17, 33, 65–66, 76
for weight loss, 39
white button, 19–20
mustard greens, 2, 15, 32, 33, 66
niacin, 10, 12, 49, 57, 74
okra, 33, 34
oleic acid, 85, 86, 96
oleuropein, 34, 84, 86
olives, 34, 84–86
omega-3s, 34, 41, 47, 50, 65, 70, 80
onions, 26–28, 33, 104
parsley, 2, 32
peas, 17, 33, 34–36, 44, 65, 66
phosphorous, 12, 37, 38, 62, 78
phytonutrients and phytochemicals, 16, 18–19, 34, 70, 74, 76
plantains, 20, 34, 65, 73–74
potassium
and bloating and constipation, 8, 9, 11–12
for bone health, 32, 33–34, 35, 38
for detoxing and cleansing, 75, 76, 79, 80
for energy, 47, 49
for heart disease, 15, 16, 20, 22
for mood boosting, 70
and salt, 8, 9, 15
for satisfying hunger, 72, 74
for the skin, 50, 52, 53, 54
for stress and tension, 2, 5
for weight loss, 41, 43
potatoes. See also sweet potatoes
for bone health, 34
for energy, 44, 47–49
for heart disease, 15, 17
for mood boosting, 65, 66
storing, 49
for stress and tension, 2
vitamins and minerals, 2, 15, 17, 34, 44, 45–49, 50, 65, 66
pregnancy, 55–59

protein, 33, 35–36, 74, 83
quercitin, 49, 90
quick-cooking veggies when you don't have time, 60–64
recipe section and symbols, 105
riboflavin, 46, 57, 58
salads and veggies, 81–86
salt, 8, 10, 12, 15, 79, 102–3
saponins, 56, 57
selenium, 25, 64, 65, 74
serotonin, 2, 5, 7, 65, 66, 67, 68, 69
shallots, 95, 104
skin dulgence, 50–54
spinach
for bone health, 32, 33, 34
cooking, 33
for detoxing and cleansing, 76
for the eyes, 64
for heart disease, 17
for mood boosting, 65, 66
for pregnancy, 55
for quick cooking, 62–64
for stress and tension, 2
vitamins and minerals, 2, 3, 17, 32, 33, 34, 55, 64, 65, 66, 76
for weight loss, 39
squash
acorn squash, 17
butternut squash, 44–47, 65
spaghetti squash, 65, 68–70, 87
for stress and tension, 2
summer squash, 2, 3–5, 8, 15, 66
vitamins and minerals, 2
winter squash, 15, 44, 45–46
yellow squash, 4
stress relieving and tension taming, 2–7
string beans, 2, 6–7, 15, 39
sweet potatoes
for bone health, 34
for heart disease, 15, 17
for mood boosting, 66–68
for pregnancy, 55

for stress and tension, 2

vitamins and minerals, 2, 15, 17, 34, 55, 66–68

Swiss chard, 15, 21–23, 32–33, 76

10-day weight loss jumpstart, belly de-bloat, and toxin flush, 240–46

thiamin, 49, 57, 58

tofu, 2, 32

tomatoes and tomato products, 2, 8, 15, 32, 33–34, 50–52, 66

tryptophan, 2, 7, 69

turnip greens

for bone health, 32, 33, 36–38

for heart disease, 15

for mood boosting, 65, 66

preparing and cooking, 38

for stress and tension, 2

vitamins and minerals, 2, 15, 32, 33, 37, 38, 65, 66

for weight loss, 39

vegetable broths, 103

veggie combos

bell peppers and spinach, 94

broccoli and tomatoes, 95–96

leeks and greens, 94–95

onions and rhubarb, 95

tomatoes and avocados, 93–94, 96

veggies to satisfy hunger, 71–74

Vitamin A

for detoxing and cleansing, 80

for energy, 47

for mood boosting, 65

for pregnancy, 55, 56, 58

in salads, 86

for skin and vision, 36, 51, 52

Vitamin B6

for cancer, 28

for detoxing and cleansing, 80

for energy, 46, 48–49

for heart disease, 16–17, 25

for mood boosting, 65, 66, 68, 69

for pregnancy, 57, 58

for satisfying hunger, 74

for stress and tension, 2

Vitamin C

for bloating and constipation, 10

for bone health, 37

boosts the immune system, 36

for cancer, 28

for detoxing and cleansing, 78, 80

for energy, 49, 50–51

for mood boosting, 65, 66, 67, 68, 69

for pregnancy, 55, 57, 58

in salads, 84

for satisfying hunger, 72

for the skin, 50, 54

for stress and tension, 2, 3, 6–7

for weight loss, 42

Vitamin D, 32, 33, 65–66, 74

Vitamin E, 55, 57, 65, 80, 86

Vitamin K

for bone health, 32, 33, 35, 37

for detoxing and cleansing, 80

for satisfying hunger, 72

for the skin, 54

for weight loss, 41, 43

Vitamins B

for energy, 47

for heart disease, 15, 16–17, 20

for pregnancy, 55, 57

in salads, 83

for satisfying hunger, 72, 74

for the skin, 54, 55

for stress and tension, 4, 6–7

for weight loss, 43

watercress, 2, 32, 33, 39–43

weight-loss veggies, 39–43

zeaxanthin, 5, 70, 83, 90

zinc, 5, 19, 21, 35, 74

zucchini, 4, 76, 158